The
Gheranda Samhita

The
Gheranda Samhita

The Original Sanskrit

and

An English Translation
James Mallinson

YogaVidya.com

An important message to our readers:

The asanas in this book should not be attempted without the supervision of an experienced teacher or prior experience. Many of the other practices should not be attempted at all. The ideas expressed in this book should not be used to diagnose, prescribe, treat, cure, or prevent any disease, illness, or individual health problem. Consult your health care practitioner for individual health care. YogaVidya.com LLC shall not be liable for any direct, indirect, incidental, special, consequential, or punitive damages resulting from the use of this book.

YogaVidya.com, PO Box 569, Woodstock NY 12498-0569 USA

YogaVidya.com and *Read the Originals* are trademarks of YogaVidya.com LLC

Printed on acid-free paper

First edition

British Library Cataloguing in Publication Data.
A catalogue record for this book is available from the British Library.

Publisher's Cataloging-in-Publication Data

Mallinson, James.
    The Gheranda Samhita: the original Sanskrit / and an English translation [by] James Mallinson.
    Woodstock, NY : YogaVidya.com, 2004.
    xvi, [128] p. : ill. ; cm.
    Includes Sanskrit and English.
ISBN 0-9716466-2-7 (hardcover)
ISBN 0-9716466-3-5 (paperback)
1. Hatha Yoga. 2. Kundalini. I. Title. II. Mallinson, James, 1970-, *tr.*
RA781.7.G43   2004
613.7'046—dc21   2004112200

Loretta made this whole deal possible.

For Sri Ram Balak Das Ji Yogiraj

Contents

Introduction

THE BOOK you are about to read, a manual of Yoga taught by Gheranda to Chanda, is the most encyclopedic of all the root texts of Hatha Yoga. At the beginning of the book, Chanda asks Gheranda to tell him about the Yoga of the body, which is the cause of knowledge of the Ultimate Reality. Gheranda assents and the book is thus called the *Gheranda Samhita*, or "The Collection [of Verses] of Gheranda."

It sets itself apart from other books on Hatha Yoga in two notable ways. Firstly, it calls its Yoga "ghata Yoga" or "ghatastha Yoga" and not Hatha Yoga. The usual meaning of ghata is "pot," but here it refers to the body, or rather the person, since the techniques taught by Gheranda work on both the body and the mind. Secondly, it is unique in teaching a sevenfold path to perfection of the person. A few Hatha Yoga texts replicate Patanjali's classical description of Yoga as ashtanga, or "eight limbed," but there are numerous other classifications. For example, the *Hatha Yoga Pradipika*'s four chapters correspond to the four stages of its Yoga, while the *Goraksha Samhita*, echoing several earlier Tantric texts, describes its Yoga as six limbed.

The seven chapters correspond to the seven means of perfecting the person. Each chapter teaches a group of techniques that, when mastered, will lead to one of the seven means listed in verse 1.9. The first chapter describes six types of cleansing techniques by which purification, the first means to perfecting the person, can be achieved. The second chapter describes thirty-two asanas by which strength, the second means, is attained. In the third chapter Gheranda teaches twenty-five mudras, which lead to steadiness, the third means. The fourth chapter describes five techniques for pratyahara, which brings about calmness, the fourth means. The fifth chapter starts with instructions on where the yogi should live, what he or she should eat, and at what time of year yogic practice should be started. It then lists ten kinds of pranayama, the practice of which leads to lightness, the fifth means. The sixth chapter describes three types of dhyana, using which the yogi can achieve realization of the self, the sixth means. Finally, in the seventh chapter, Gheranda teaches six types of samadhi, which lead to abstraction, the ultimate means of perfecting the person.[1]

Like the other root texts of Hatha Yoga, the *Gheranda Samhita* does not concern itself with yama and niyama, the restraints and observances that make up the first two limbs of classical Yoga. It is unique in devoting an entire chapter

---

[1]In verse 7.6, it is said that Raja Yoga is of six types. Many commentators equate Raja Yoga with the classical Yoga of Patanjali's *Yoga Sutras*, but in texts on Hatha Yoga it means samadhi, rather than a separate type of Yoga.

to bodily purification and in the number of purificatory practices it describes. The chapters on asanas and mudras are similarly unparalleled in the number of practices taught. The difference between asanas and mudras is not made clear by Gheranda—several of the mudras seem to be no more than asanas. We are told in the first chapter that asanas lead to strength and mudras to steadiness. In other texts, however, the purpose of mudras is said to be the awakening of Kundalini. In five of the twenty-five mudras listed this aim is made explicit, but awakening of the Goddess is also given as one of the fruits of pranayama in verse 5.57.

A further unique aspect of this book lies in its positioning of the chapter on pratyahara before that on pranayama. In the classical system, the last six limbs are successively more subtle, moving from the physical realm to the mental. Pranayama is, of course, a more physical practice than pratyahara, but here the Bhramari pranayama is said to lead to samadhi; indeed, it is one of the six varieties of Raja Yoga or samadhi given in the final chapter. This may account for the position of the chapter on pranayama. Most of the rest of the chapter is similar to other texts, apart from the teaching of the Ajapa Gayatri, the mantra constantly but involuntarily repeated by all living beings. The sounds of the in- and out-breaths are said to be *sa* and *ham*, whose implicit combination is the Vedantic dictum *so'ham*, "I am that."

The chapter on dhyana teaches three successively more subtle visualizations, starting with a gross dhyana of the yogi's guru on a beautiful island, followed by a luminous dhyana, visualization of a light between the eyebrows, and a subtle dhyana, visualization of Kundalini. In the final chapter Gheranda teaches six very different ways to samadhi. Three mudras, Shambhavi, Khechari, and Yoni, lead to three types of samadhi: dhyana, bliss through rasa ("taste" or "sensation"), and laya (resorption into the Ultimate Reality by means of Kundalini's rise up the Sushumna, or central channel). Bhramari pranayama, as noted above, leads to samadhi through nada, the inner sound. The Murccha, or "trance" pranayama also leads to samadhi. Finally, we are told that samadhi can arise through bhakti, "devotion," and this is another feature that sets this book apart from all other texts on Hatha Yoga.

Nothing is known about Gheranda and Chanda. The name Gheranda is not found anywhere else in Sanskrit literature. Like many other works on Hatha Yoga, the work is framed as a dialogue, suggesting that it has been overheard and then written down. Thus the identity of the author (or whoever overheard Gheranda) is not revealed. Chanda's full name, Chandakapali, means "fierce skullbearer." The epithet kapali, "skullbearer," immediately brings to mind the sect of the Kapalikas, skull-bearing followers of Shiva infamous for antinomian practices. Kapali and Kapalika are both mentioned as past masters of Hatha Yoga in the list given in verses 1.4-8 of the *Hatha Yoga Pradipika*. (In fact, some manuscripts of the *Hatha Yoga Pradipika* prefix the name Kapali with Chanda, rather than Khanda, the more common reading.) However, as we shall see below, the practices taught in this book are tame compared to some of those taught in other works on Hatha Yoga, and Gheranda appears to have been a follower of Vishnu, so we cannot claim Kapalika origins for the text. Perhaps Chanda's epithet is simply a way of establishing a connection between the text and the lineage of the Mahasiddhas mentioned in the *Hatha Yoga Pradipika*.

There are also no records of the place and date of composition of the text, but there are indications that it is a relatively late work on Hatha Yoga from northeast India. The majority of its manuscripts are found in the north and east of India, and, of those which are dated, the oldest was copied in Bengal in 1802 C.E. As far as I am aware, it was never cited by medieval commentators in their works on Hatha Yoga. Doctrinal discontinuities also set it apart from the rest of the Hatha Yogic corpus. Tantric influences have been toned down considerably. See, for example, the description of Vajrolimudra in verse 3.39: in all other manuals of Hatha Yoga this name is given to a technique in which the yogi or yogini resorbs commingled sexual fluids through the urethra; here it is a simple physical posture. The author attributes the teachings of Hatha Yoga to Shiva, but verses 5.77 and 7.18 suggest that he was a devotee of Vishnu. Furthermore, several verses indicate that the text was compiled by a vedantin, in particular verse 7.4: "I am Brahman and nothing else. I am Brahman alone and do not suffer. My form is truth, consciousness, and bliss. I am eternally free. I abide in my own nature."[2]

---

[2]Despite the author's sectarian affiliation, he has no particular doctrinal axe to grind and often tells the aspiring yogi to fill in the details of his visualizations and practices in the manner instructed by his guru.

The early texts of Hatha Yoga showed no trace of Vedanta; their doctrinal framework was Tantric. As Hatha Yoga and its proponents, the Nathas, gained in popularity and patronage, the religious orthodox, amongst whom Vedanta had become the predominant ideology, had to sit up and take notice. As they had done with other heterodox movements that threatened their hegemony (e.g., renunciation and vegetarianism) they claimed Hatha Yoga as their own. This process culminated in the eighteenth century with the compilation of several new Upanishads and the rewriting of some older ones; these are now known collectively as the Yoga Upanishads. The unknown compiler(s) used verses from established works on Hatha Yoga to create the texts. The Vedantic and Vaishnava leanings in this book, combined with its use of verses from established works on Hatha Yoga, suggest that it probably resulted from a similar process. In the light of this, as well as the fact that errors in the manuscript of 1802 C.E. imply an established manuscript tradition, the absence of citations in seventeenth-century commentaries, and the location of most of its manuscripts in Bengal, we may hazard a guess that the *Gheranda Samhita* was composed in Bengal around 1700 C.E.

The Sanskrit text presented here is based on the edition of Swami Digambarji and Dr. M. L. Gharote, first published at Lonavala, Maharashtra, in 1978, for which they collated fourteen manuscripts and five printed books, including the Adyar Library edition of 1933, which formed the foundation of their edition. The best known edition of the text is that of Chandra Vasu, which was first published in 1915. It was based on two earlier Bengali editions which appear to have relied on a very small number of manuscripts. The Adyar Library edition is much more thorough and omits several spurious verses found in Vasu's edition. I consulted three manuscripts (two in the library in Jodhpur's Mehrangarh Fort and one in the Bodleian Library, Oxford) that were not collated for the Lonavala edition, but they were very similar to manuscripts that had been used so I decided that there was no point in editing the text myself. I have made emendations or adopted alternative readings in a few places, but in general the text is the same as the Lonavala edition.[3] The Sanskrit is of the variety that medieval commentators on Tantric and Yogic works generously called "aisha," which literally means "coming from Shiva." In other words, it is often ungrammatical.

Some verses have been borrowed from other works, in particular the *Hatha Yoga Pradipika* and the *Goraksha Samhita*. The section on the five dharanas (elemental visualizations) in verses 3.59-63 sheds light on the text's composition and development. It has clearly been taken directly from the *Goraksha Samhita*, verses 155-59, but is incoherent and ungrammatical in all the *Gheranda Samhita* manuscripts. In the *Goraksha Samhita* each element has a

---

[3]These critical editions are mentioned in the introduction and footnotes. The first work has been referred to as the *Goraksha Samhita*.

Nowotny, Fausta. Das Gorakṣaśataka. Dokumente der Geistesgeschichte 3. Köln: K. A. Nowotny, 1976.

Digambarji, Swami, and Dr. M. L. Gharote, eds. Gheraṇḍsaṃhitā. Lonāvalā: Kaivalyadhāma Śrīman Mādhav Yoga Mandir Samiti, 1978.

Mallik, Kalyani. The Siddhasiddhāntapaddhati and Other Works of Nātha Yogīs. Poona: Oriental Book House, 1954.

color, a shape, a location in the body, and a mantra, but these are confused and omitted in the *Gheranda Samhita*. In verse 3.62, for example, the wind element is said to be black, smoky, and white, while in the *Goraksha Samhita* it is just black. I have somewhat boldly decided to adopt the readings of the *Goraksha Samhita* for the entire passage. That all the *Gheranda Samhita* manuscripts present a similarly incoherent description of the dharanas is surprising and points to two possible scenarios. Either they are descended from a single flawed manuscript or the compiler of the *Gheranda Samhita* was using a flawed manuscript of the *Goraksha Samhita* to write the text. The first hypothesis requires a lengthy and improbably irregular manuscript tradition predating the earliest extant manuscript, which, in the absence of external evidence for the text's existence prior to 1802 C.E., is unlikely. I am thus inclined to believe the second hypothesis.

In translating, I have tried to be as literal as possible without sacrificing readability. I have sought not to add anything to what is found in the Sanskrit text—commentary and elucidation are for the practitioner's guru. Thus where the instructions for a practice are ambiguous, they have been left that way. The photographs of the asanas and mudras draw from the descriptions in the text. In a few instances those descriptions do not provide all the information necessary to be sure of the correct posture. For those cases I have relied on current practice and common sense to fill in the gaps.

Purification

एकदा चण्डकापालिर्गत्वा घेरण्डकुट्टिरम् ।
प्रणम्य विनयाद्भक्त्या घेरण्डं परिपृच्छति ॥ १
घटस्थयोगं योगेश तत्त्वज्ञानस्य कारणम् ।
इदानीं श्रोतुमिच्छामि योगेश्वर वद प्रभो ॥ २

One day Chanda the Skullbearer went to Gheranda's
hut. After bowing politely he humbly asked of Gheranda,
"King of Yoga, I now want to hear about the Yoga of the
body, the cause of knowledge of the Ultimate Reality.
Lord of Yoga, speak, O master!"

साधु साधु महाबाहो यन्मां त्वं परिपृच्छसि ।
कथयामि हि ते वत्स सावधानोऽवधारय ॥ ३

"You have done very well indeed in asking me this. I shall
certainly tell you, my child. Listen carefully.

नास्ति मायासमः पाशो नास्ति योगात्परं बलम् ।
नास्ति ज्ञानात्परो बन्धुर्नाहंकारात्परो रिपुः ॥ ४

1

There is no fetter like illusion, no force greater than Yoga, no friend greater than knowledge, and no enemy greater than ego.

अभ्यासात्कादिवर्णानां यथा शास्त्राणि बोधयेत् ।
तथा योगं समासाद्य तत्त्वज्ञानं च लभ्यते ॥ ५

Just as from studying the alphabet one may understand the scriptural teachings, so by practicing Yoga one may obtain knowledge of the Ultimate Reality.

सुकृतैर्दुष्कृतैर्कार्यैर्जायते प्राणिनां घटः ।
घटादुत्पद्यते कर्म घटीयन्त्रं यथा भ्रमेत् ॥ ६

The bodies of living beings are created by their good and bad deeds; action is born of the body. Thus the noria turns.[1]

ऊर्ध्वाधो भ्रमते यद्वद्घटीयन्त्रं गवां वशात् ।
तद्वत्कर्मवशाज्जीवो भ्रमते जन्ममृत्युभिः ॥ ७

In the same way that the noria revolves up and down, driven by cows, so, driven by action, the jiva wanders through births and deaths.[2]

आमकुम्भ इवाम्भःस्थो जीर्यमाणः सदा घटः ।

---

[1] A noria is a wheel fitted with buckets to lift water for irrigation.
[2] Jiva or jivatman is used to describe the soul when it is animating a living body.

योगानलेन संदह्य घटशुद्धिं समाचरेत् ॥ ८

Like an unbaked pot in water, the body is always decaying. One should bake it with the fire of Yoga and make it pure.

शोधनं दृढता चैव स्थैर्यं धैर्यं च लाघवम् ।
प्रत्यक्षं च निर्लिप्तं च घटस्य सप्तसाधनम् ॥ ९

Purification, strength, steadiness, calmness, lightness, realization, and abstraction are the seven means of perfecting the body.

षट्कर्मणा शोधनं च आसनेन भवेद्दृढम् ।
मुद्रया स्थिरता चैव प्रत्याहारेण धीरता ॥ १०

The six cleansing techniques bring about purification and asanas bring about strength; mudras bring about steadiness and pratyahara brings about calmness.

प्राणायामाल्लाघवं च ध्यानात्प्रत्यक्षमात्मनः ।
समाधिना निर्लिप्तं च मुक्तिरेव न संशयः ॥ ११

From pranayama, lightness arises and from dhyana, realization of the self. Through samadhi arises abstraction and liberation itself; in this there is no doubt.

धौतिर्बस्तिस्तथा नेतिर्नौलिकी त्राटकं तथा ।
कपालभातिश्चैतानि षट्कर्माणि समाचरेत् ॥ १२

Dhauti, Basti, Neti, Nauli, Trataka, and Kapalabhati; one should practice these six cleansing techniques.

अन्तर्धौतिर्दन्तधौतिर्हृद्धौतिर्मूलशोधनम् ।
धौत्यश्चतुर्विधाः प्रोक्ता घटं कुर्वन्ति निर्मलम् ॥ 13

The four types of dhauti are called Antardhauti, Danta-dhauti, Hriddhauti, and Mulashodhana. They clean the body.

वातसारं वारिसारं वह्निसारं बहिष्कृतम् ।
घटस्य निर्मलार्थाय ह्यन्तर्धौतिश्चतुर्विधा ॥ 14

Vatasara, Varisara, Vahnisara, and Bahishkrita are the four types of antardhauti used to clean the body.

काकचञ्चुवदास्येन पिबेद्वायुं शनैः शनैः ।
चालयेदुदरं पश्चाद्वर्त्मना रेचयेच्छनैः ॥ 15

With the mouth like a crow's beak, inhale very slowly, move the stomach, and then slowly expel the air through the lower passage.

वातसारं परं गोप्यं देहनिर्मलकारकम् ।
सर्वरोगक्षयकरं देहानलविवर्धकम् ॥ 16

The great Vatasara is to be kept secret. It cleans the body, destroys all diseases, and increases the body's fire.

आकण्ठं पूरयेद्वारि वक्त्रेण च पिबेच्छनैः ।
चाल्येदुदरेणैव चोदरादेच्चयेदधः ॥ 17

Slowly drink water through the mouth until full up to the throat. Move it through the stomach and expel it from the stomach downwards.

वारिसारं परं गोप्यं देहनिर्मलकारकम् ।
साधयेद्यः प्रयत्नेन देवदेहं प्रपद्यते ॥ 18

The great Varisara is to be kept secret. It cleans the body. The yogi who practices it zealously obtains a divine body.

नाभिग्रन्थिं मेरुपृष्ठे शतवारं च कारयेत् ।
उदर्यमामयं त्यक्त्वा जाठराग्निं विवर्धयेत् ॥ 19

Move the navel plexus to the spinal column one hundred times. This gets rid of intestinal diseases and increases the digestive fire.

वह्निसारमियं धौतिर्योगिनां योगसिद्धिदा ।
एषा धौतिः परा गोप्या न प्रकाश्या कदाचन ॥ 20

This Vahnisara dhauti brings about success in Yoga for yogis. This great dhauti is to be kept secret and never revealed.

काकीमुद्रां साधयित्वा पूरयेदुदरं मरुत् ।

धारयेदर्धयामं तु चालयेदधवर्त्मना ॥ 21

Fill the stomach with air using Kakimudra. Hold it for ninety minutes and move it through the lower passage.

नाभिदघ्ने जले स्थित्वा शक्तिनाडीं विसर्जयेत् ।
कराभ्यां क्षालयेन्नाडीं यावन्मलविसर्जनम् ।
तावत्प्रक्षाल्य नाडीं च उदरे वेशयेत्पुनः ॥ 22

Standing in water up to the navel, draw out the shakti nadi. Wash the nadi with both hands until the dirt has come out, then rinse it and put it back in the stomach.

इदं प्रक्षालनं गोप्यं देवानामपि दुर्लभम् ।
केवलं धौतिमात्रेण देवदेहो भवेद्ध्रुवम् ॥ 23

This washing is to be kept secret; it is difficult for even the gods to attain. It is certainly only by dhauti alone that a divine body may arise.

यामार्धधारणाशक्तिं यावन्न साधयेन्नरः ।
बहिष्कृतं महाधौतिं तावन्नैव समाचरेत् ॥ 24

Until a man is able to hold his breath for ninety minutes, he must not practice the great Bahishkritadhauti.

दन्तमूलं जिह्वामूलं रन्ध्रे च कर्णयुग्मयोः ।
कपालरन्ध्रं पञ्चैते दन्तधौतिर्विधीयते ॥ 25

The base of the teeth, the base of the tongue, in the openings of each of the ears, and the cranial aperture: Dantadhauti is divided into these five types.

खादिरेण रसेनाथ मृत्तिकया च शुद्धया ।
मार्जयेद्दन्तमूलं च यावत्किल्बिषमाहरेत् ॥ 26

Using acacia resin or clean earth, rub the base of the teeth until the impurities are removed.

दन्तमूलं परा धौतिर्योगिनां योगसाधने ।
नित्यं कुर्यात्प्रभाते च दन्तरक्षाय योगवित् ।
दन्तमूलं धावनादिकार्येषु योगिनां मतम् ॥ 27

Cleaning the base of the teeth is an important dhauti in the Yoga practice of yogis; in order to look after his teeth, the knower of Yoga should do it every morning. The cleaning of the base of the teeth is considered to be one of the essential cleansing processes for yogis.

अथातः संप्रवक्ष्यामि जिह्वाशोधनकारणम् ।
जरामरणरोगादीन्नाशयेद्दीर्घलम्बिका ॥ 28

Now I shall teach the technique for cleaning the tongue. A long tongue can get rid of old age, death, disease, and the like.[3]

_____

[3] A long tongue can do this because it enables the yogi to perform Khechari-mudra. See verses 3.21–28.

तर्जनीमध्यमानामा अङ्गुलित्रययोगतः ।
वेशयेद्गलमध्ये तु मार्जयेल्लम्बिकामूलम् ।
शनैः शनैर्मार्जयित्वा कफदोषं निवारयेत् ॥ 29

Join together the index, middle, and ring fingers,
put them into the throat and rub clean the root of the
tongue. By very gentle rubbing the yogi can prevent
imbalances of kapha.[4]

मार्जयेन्नवनीतेन दोहयेच्च पुनः पुनः ।
तदग्रं लोहयन्त्रेण कर्षयित्वा पुनः पुनः ॥ 30

After repeatedly pulling its tip with iron tongs, rub it with
fresh butter and milk it over and over again.

नित्यं कुर्यात्प्रयत्नेन रवेरुदयकेऽस्तके ।
एवं कृते च नित्यं सा लम्बिका दीर्घतां व्रजेत् ॥ 31

Do this carefully every day at sunrise and sunset. When
regularly done in this way, the tongue becomes long.

तर्जन्यङ्गुल्यकाग्रेण मार्जयेत्कर्णरन्ध्रयोः ।
नित्यमभ्यासयोगेन नादान्तरं प्रकाशयेत् ॥ 32

Using the tip of the index finger, rub clean the apertures of
the ears. By regular practice the inner sound will manifest.

---

[4]Kapha is one of the three doshas, or humors, of Ayurveda, and may be compared
to phlegm. The other two are pitta (bile) and vata (wind).

वृद्धाङ्गुष्ठेन दक्षेण मर्दयेद्धालरन्ध्रकम् ।
एवमभ्यासयोगेन कफदोषं निवारयेत् ॥ 33

With the right thumb, rub the aperture at the roof of the
mouth. By practicing thus one can prevent imbalances
of kapha.

नाडी निर्मलतां याति दिव्यदृष्टिः प्रजायते ।
निद्रान्ते भोजनान्ते च दिवान्ते च दिने दिने ॥ 34

The nadis become clean and divine sight arises. It should
be done daily: on waking, after food, and at the end
of the day.

हृद्धौतिं त्रिविधां कुर्याद्दण्डवमनवाससा ॥ 35

The yogi should practice three types of hriddhauti: with a
stick, by vomiting, and with a cloth.

रम्भादण्डं हरिद्दण्डं वेत्रदण्डं तथैव च ।
हन्मध्ये चालयित्वा तु पुनः प्रत्याहरेच्छनैः ॥ 36

Insert a stick of plantain, turmeric, or cane into the gullet,
move it about, and then slowly withdraw it.

कफं पित्तं तथा क्लेदं रेचयेदूर्ध्ववर्त्मना ।
दण्डधौतिविधानेन हृद्रोगं नाशयेद्ध्रुवम् ॥ 37

One thus ejects phlegm, bile, and slime through the upper passage. By using the Dandadhauti technique, one is sure to eliminate diseases of the throat.

भोजनान्ते पिबेद्वारि चाकण्ठं पूरितं सुधीः ।
ऊर्ध्वां दृष्टिं क्षणं कृत्वा तज्जलं वमयेत्पुनः ।
नित्यमभ्यासयोगेन कफपित्तं निवारयेत् ॥ ३८

When he has finished eating, the wise man should drink water until he is full up to his throat. After looking upwards for a moment, he should vomit the water. By regularly using this practice he prevents imbalances of kapha and pitta.

चतुरङ्गुलविस्तारं सूक्ष्मवस्त्रं शनैर्ग्रसेत् ।
पुनः प्रत्याहरेदेतत्प्रोच्यते धौतिकर्मकम् ॥ ३९

Slowly swallow a piece of fine cloth four fingers wide and then withdraw it. This technique is called Dhauti.

गुल्मज्वरप्लीहाकुष्ठकफपित्तं विनश्यति ।
आरोग्यं बलपुष्टिश्च भवेत्तस्य दिने दिने ॥ ४०

Intestinal tumors, fever, diseases of the spleen, skin ailments, and imbalances of kapha and pitta are destroyed. One becomes healthier and stronger every day.

अपानक्रूरता तावद्यावन्मूलं न शोधयेत् ।

तस्मात्सर्वप्रयत्नेन मूलशोधनमाचरेत् ॥ ४१

Until the yogi cleans his rectum he will have difficulties with wind. Therefore he should practice Mulashodhana to the best of his ability.

पीतमूलस्य दण्डेन मध्यमाङ्गुलिनापि वा ।
यत्नेन क्षालयेद्गुह्यं वारिणा च पुनः पुनः ॥ ४२

With the help of either a stick of turmeric or the middle finger, carefully and repeatedly wash the rectum with water.

वारयेत्कोष्ठकाठिन्यमामाजीर्णं निवारयेत् ।
कारणं कान्तिपुष्ट्योश्च वह्निमण्डलदीपनम् ॥ ४३

This keeps intestinal problems at bay and prevents the buildup of undigested matter. It brings about beauty and health and kindles the digestive fire.

जलबस्तिः शुष्कबस्तिर्बस्ती च द्विविधौ स्मृतौ ।
जलबस्तिं जले कुर्याच्छुष्कबस्तिं क्षितौ सदा ॥ ४४

Basti is said to be of two kinds: wet and dry. One should always practice wet Basti in water and dry Basti on land.

नाभिदघ्ने जले पायुन्यस्तनालोत्कटासनः ।
आकुञ्चनं प्रकाशं च जलबस्तिं समाचरेत् ॥ ४५

Squatting in water up to the navel with a pipe inserted in the anus, practice wet Basti by contraction and dilation.

प्रमेहं च गुदावर्तं क्रूरवायुं निवारयेत् ।
भवेत्स्वच्छन्ददेहश्च कामदेवसमो भवेत् ॥ 46

One keeps urinary diseases, constipation, and problems with wind at bay, and becomes like the God of Love, with a body of one's own choosing.

पश्चिमोत्तानतो बस्तिं चालयित्वा शनैरधः ।
अश्विनीमुद्रया पायुमाकुञ्चयेत्प्रकाशयेत् ॥ 47

Assuming Paschimottanasana, very gently move the abdominal area and then contract and dilate the anus with Ashvinimudra.

एवमभ्यासयोगेन कोष्ठदोषो न विद्यते ।
विवर्धयेज्जाठराग्निमामवातं विनाशयेत् ॥ 48

By practicing thus, intestinal ailments do not arise. One increases the digestive fire and eliminates constipation and wind.

वितस्तिमानं सूक्ष्मसूत्रं नासानाले प्रवेशयेत् ।
मुखान्निर्गमयेत्पश्चात्प्रोच्यते नेतिकर्मकम् ॥ 49

Insert a thin thread nine inches long into the nostril and then draw it out of the mouth. This technique is called Neti.

साधनान्नेतिकार्यस्य खेचरीसिद्धिमाप्नुयात् ।
कफदोषा विनश्यन्ति दिव्यदृष्टिः प्रजायते ॥ 50

By practicing Neti, one can master Khechari. Imbalances
of kapha disappear and divine sight arises.

अमन्दवेगेन तुन्दं भ्रामयेदुभपाश्र्वयोः ।
सर्वरोगान्निहन्तीह देहानलविवर्धनम् ॥ 51

Rotate the stomach quickly on both sides.[5] This gets rid
of all diseases and the bodily fire increases.

निमेषोन्मेषकं त्यक्त्वा सूक्ष्मलक्ष्यं निरीक्षयेत् ।
पतन्ति यावदश्रूणि त्राटकं प्रोच्यते बुधैः ॥ 52

Stare at a small object without blinking until tears start to
fall. The wise call this Trataka.

एवमभ्यासयोगेन शाम्भवी जायते ध्रुवम् ।
नेत्ररोगा विनश्यन्ति दिव्यदृष्टिः प्रजायते ॥ 53

By using this practice, Shambhavi is sure to arise.[6]
Diseases of the eye disappear; one gets divine sight.

वातक्रमेण व्युत्क्रमेण शीत्क्रमेण विशेषतः ।
भालभातिं त्रिधा कुर्यात्कफदोषं निवारयेत् ॥ 54

---

[5]This is Nauli.
[6]Shambhavimudra is described in verses 3.53–56.

One should practice Bhalabhati in three ways—with Vatakrama, Vyutkrama, or Shitkrama—and keep imbalances of kapha at bay.[7]

इडया पूरयेद्वायुं रेचयेत्पिङ्गलया पुनः ।
पिङ्गलया पूरयित्वा पुनश्चन्द्रेण रेचयेत् ॥ 55

Inhale through the left nostril and then exhale through the right. Then, after filling yourself up with air by inhaling through the right nostril, exhale through the left.

पूरकं रेचकं कृत्वा वेगेन न तु धारयेत् ।
एवमभ्यासयोगेन कफदोषं निवारयेत् ॥ 56

Inhale and exhale quickly and do not hold the breath. By using this practice one keeps imbalances of kapha at bay.

नासाभ्यां जलमाकृष्य पुनर्वक्त्रेण रेचयेत् ।
पायं पायं व्युत्क्रमेण श्लेष्मदोषं निवारयेत् ॥ 57

Draw in water through the nostrils and then expel it through the mouth. Repeated drinking by means of Vyutkrama keeps imbalances of kapha at bay.

शीत्कृत्य पीत्वा वक्त्रेण नासानलैर्विरेचयेत् ।

---

[7]Bhalabhati and Kapalabhati are two different names for the same practice. Bhati literally means "luster." The implication is that the skull (kapala) or forehead (bhala) will shine as a result of this practice.

एवमभ्यासयोगेन कामदेवसमो भवेत् ॥ 58

Drink water through the mouth with a slurping sound and expel it through the nostrils. By using this practice one becomes like the God of Love.

न जायते वार्द्धकं च ज्वरो नैव प्रजायते ।
भवेत्स्वच्छन्ददेहश्च कफदोषं निवारयेत् ॥ 59

One does not grow old, one does not get fevers, one has whatever body one wishes for, and one keeps imbalances of kapha at bay.

इति श्रीघेरण्डसंहितायां घेरण्डचण्डसंवादे
घटस्थयोगे षट्कर्मसाधनं नाम प्रथमोपदेशः ॥

Thus ends the first chapter, called the practice of the six cleansing techniques, in the glorious Gheranda Samhita, a dialogue between Gheranda and Chanda on bodily Yoga.

Chapter Two

Asanas

आसनानि समस्तानि यावन्तो जीवजन्तवः ।
चतुरशीति लक्षाणि शिवेन कथितानि च ॥ 1

All together there are as many asanas as there are species
of living beings. Shiva has taught 8,400,000.

तेषां मध्ये विशिष्टानि षोडशोनं शतं कृतम् ।
तेषां मध्ये मर्त्यलोके द्वात्रिंशदासनं शुभम् ॥ 2

Of these, eighty-four are preeminent, of which thirty-two
are useful in the world of mortals.

सिद्धं पद्मं तथा भद्रं मुक्तं वज्रं च स्वस्तिकम् ।
सिंहं च गोमुखं वीरं धनुरासनमेव च ॥ 3
मृतं गुप्तं तथा मात्स्यं मत्स्येन्द्रासनमेव च ।
गोरक्षं पश्चिमोत्तानमुत्कटं संकटं तथा ॥ 4
मयूरं कुक्कुटं कूर्मं तथा चोत्तानकूर्मकम् ।
उत्तानमण्डुकं वृक्षं मण्डुकं गरुडं वृषम् ॥ 5
शलभं मकरं चोष्ट्रं भुजङ्गं च योगासनम् ।

द्वात्रिंशदासनान्येव मर्त्यलोके च सिद्धिदा ॥ 6

Siddha, Padma, Bhadra, Mukta, Vajra, Svastika, Simha,
Gomukha, Vira, and Dhanur; Mrita, Gupta, Matsya,
Matsyendra, Goraksha, Paschimottana, Utkata, and
Sankata; Mayura, Kukkuta, Kurma, Uttanakurmaka,
Uttanamanduka, Vriksha, Manduka, Garuda, and Vrisha;
Shalabha, Makara, Ushtra, Bhujanga, and Yoga: these
thirty-two asanas bestow success in the world of mortals.

योनिस्थानकमङ्घ्रिमूलघटितं संपीड्य गुल्फेतरं
मेढ्रोपर्यथ संनिधाय चिबुकं कृत्वा हृदि स्थापितम् ।
स्थाणुः संयमितेन्द्रियोऽचलदृशा पश्यन्भ्रुवोरन्तरम्
एतन्मोक्षकपाटभेदनकरं सिद्धासनं प्रोच्यते ॥ 7

Press one heel against the perineum, put the other ankle
above the penis, place the chin on the chest, and remain
motionless with the sense organs restrained while staring
between the eyebrows. This is called Siddhasana and it
breaks open the door to liberation.

वामोरूपरि दक्षिणं हि चरणं संस्थाप्य वामं तथा
दक्षोरूपरि पश्चिमेन विधिना धृत्वा कराभ्यां दृढम् ।
अङ्गुष्ठौ हृदये निधाय चिबुकं नासाग्रमालोकयेद्
एतद्व्याधिविकारनाशनकरं पद्मासनं प्रोच्यते ॥ 8

Place the right foot on top of the left thigh and the left
foot on top of the right thigh, take a firm hold of the toes
with the hands from behind, place the chin on the chest,

and look at the tip of the nose. This is called Padmasana and it destroys diseases and ailments.

गुल्फौ च वृषणस्याधो व्युत्क्रमेण समाहितौ ।
पादाङ्गुष्ठौ कराभ्यां च धृत्वा वै पृष्ठदेशतः ॥ ९

Put both heels together, turn them back below the scrotum, and take hold of the toes from behind.

जालन्धरं समासाद्य नासाग्रमवलोकयेत् ।
भद्रासनं भवेदेतत्सर्वव्याधिविनाशकम् ॥ १०

Applying Jalandhara, look at the tip of the nose. This is Bhadrasana. It destroys all diseases.

पायुमूले वामगुल्फं दक्षगुल्फं तथोपरि ।
समकायशिरोग्रीवं मुक्तासनं तु सिद्धिदम् ॥ ११

Put the left heel under the anus and the right heel on top of it. Keep the body, head, and neck straight. This is Muktasana. It bestows success.

जङ्घाभ्यां वज्रवत्कृत्वा गुदपार्श्वे पदावुभौ ।
वज्रासनं भवेदेतद्योगिनां सिद्धिदायकम् ॥ १२

Make the thighs as hard as diamond and put the feet on either side of the anus. This is Vajrasana. It bestows success upon yogis.

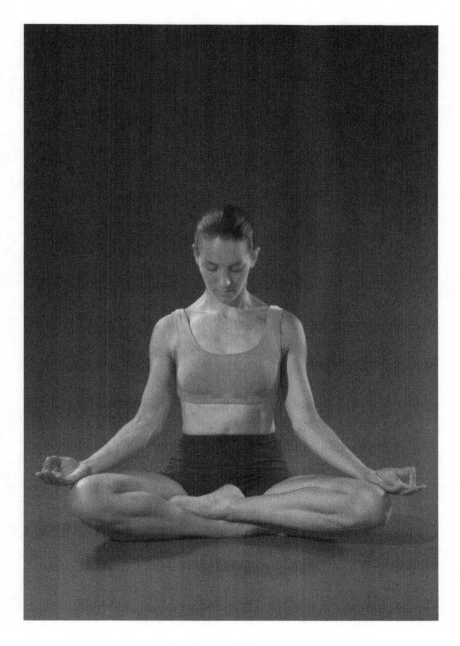

सिद्धासन – Siddhasana

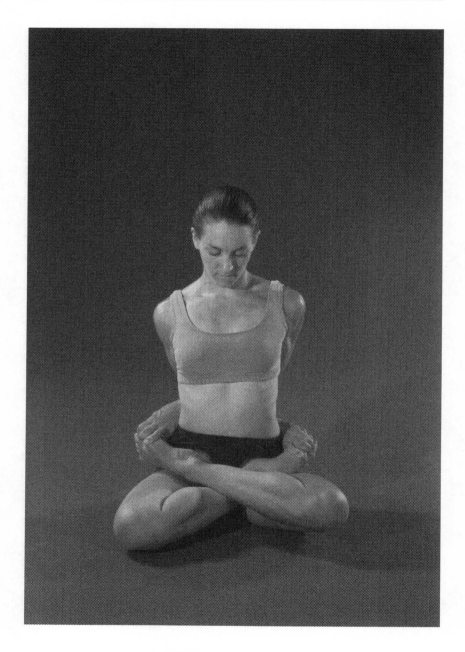

पद्मासन – Padmasana

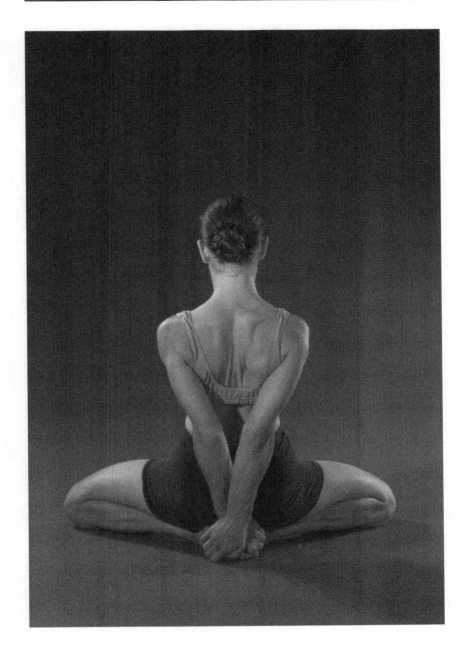

भद्रासन – Bhadrasana

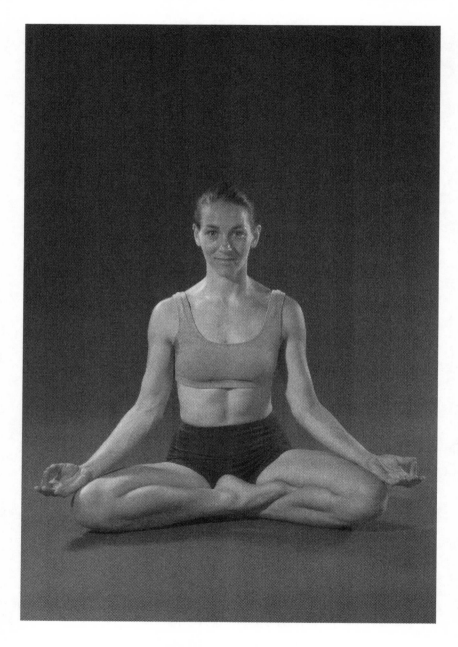

मुक्तासन – Muktasana

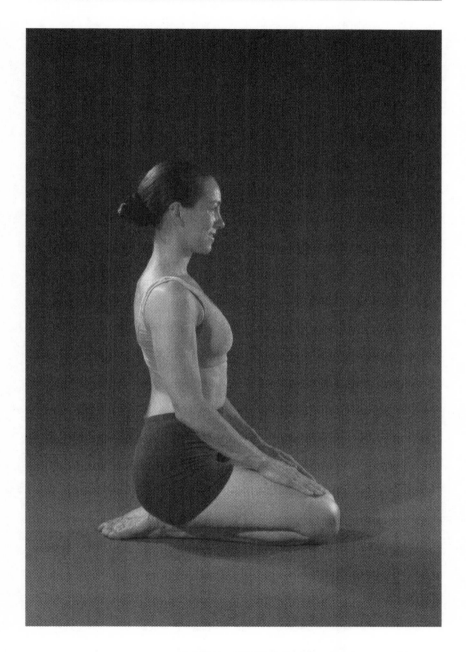

वज्रासन – Vajrasana

जानूर्वोरन्तरे कृत्वा योगी पादतले उभे ।
ऋजुकायः समासीनः स्वस्तिकं तत्प्रचक्षते ॥ 13

The yogi should put the soles of both feet between the calves and the thighs and sit with a straight body. That is called Svastikasana.

गुल्फौ च वृषणस्याधो व्युत्क्रमेणोर्ध्वतां गतौ ।
चितियुग्मं भूमिसंस्थं करौ च जानुनोपरि ॥ 14

Put both heels (crossed and turned upwards) underneath the scrotum, the shins on the ground, and the hands on top of the knees.

व्यात्तवक्त्रो जलन्धरेण नासाग्रमवलोकयेत् ।
सिंहासनं भवेदेतत्सर्वव्याधिविनाशकम् ॥ 15

Openmouthed and applying Jalandhara, look at the tip of the nose. This is Simhasana. It destroys all diseases.

पादौ च भूमौ संस्थाप्य पृष्ठपार्श्वे निवेशयेत् ।
स्थिरं कायं समासाद्य गोमुखं गोमुखाकृति ॥ 16

Place both feet on the ground, putting them on either side of the bottom, and hold the body steady. This is Gomukhasana; it looks like a cow's face.

एकं पादमथैकस्मिन्विन्यसेदूरुसंस्थितम् ।

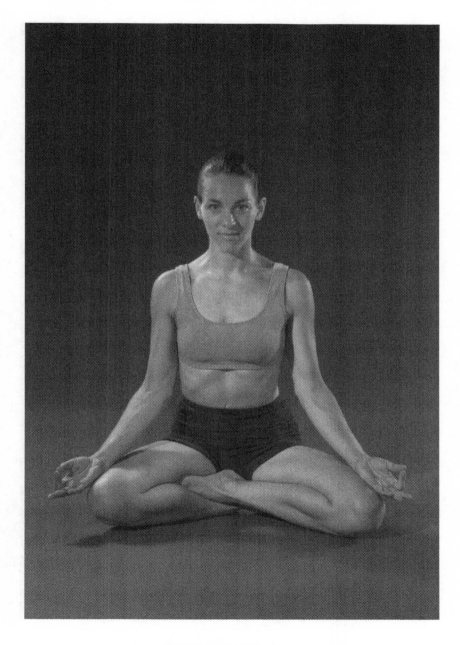

स्वस्तिकासन – Svastikasana

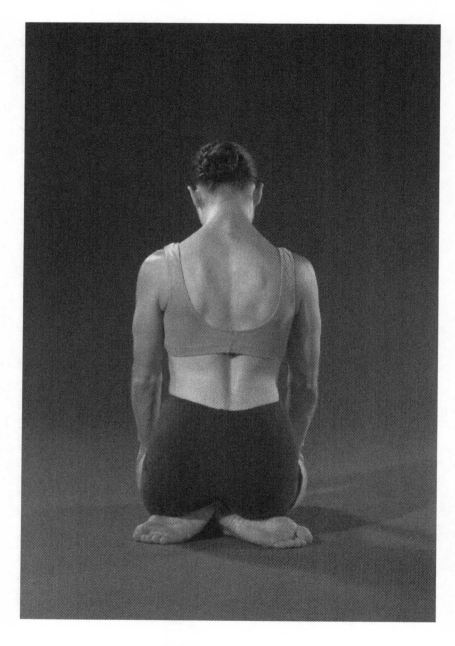

सिंहासन – Simhasana

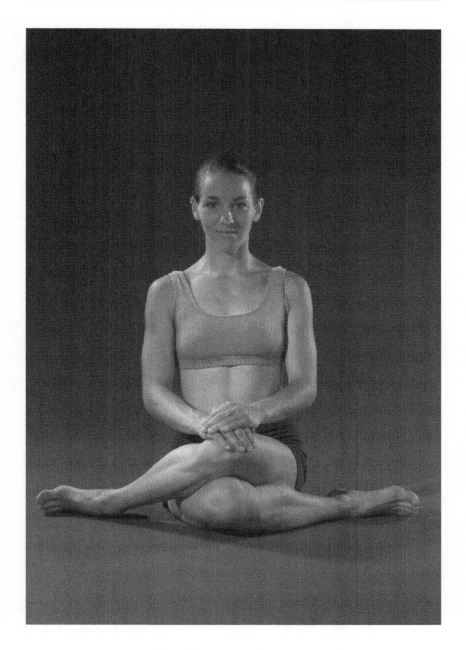

गोमुखासन – Gomukhasana

इतरस्मिंस्तथा पश्चाद्वीरासनमितीरितम् ॥ 17

Place one foot on one thigh and then the other foot under the same thigh. This is called Virasana.

प्रसार्य पादौ भुवि दण्डरूपौ करौ च पृष्ठे धृतपादयुग्मं ।
कृत्वा धनुर्वत्परिवर्तिताङ्गं निगद्यते वै धनुरासनं तत् ॥ 18

Stretch the legs out on the ground like a stick, extend the arms, hold both feet from behind with the hands, and make the body curved like a bow. That is called Dhanurasana.

उत्तानं शववद्भूमौ शयानं तु शवासनम् ।
शवासनं श्रमहरं चित्तविश्रान्तिकारणम् ॥ 19

Lying stretched out on the ground like a corpse is Shavasana.[1] Shavasana removes fatigue and brings rest to the mind.

जानुर्वोरन्तरे पादौ कृत्वा पादौ च गोपयेत् ।
पादोपरि च संस्थाप्य गुदं गुप्तासनं विदुः ॥ 20

Conceal the feet between the calves and the thighs and put the anus on top of them. This is known as Guptasana.

मुक्तपद्मासनं कृत्वा उत्तानशयनं चरेत् ।

---

[1]Shavasana and Mritasana are synonyms.

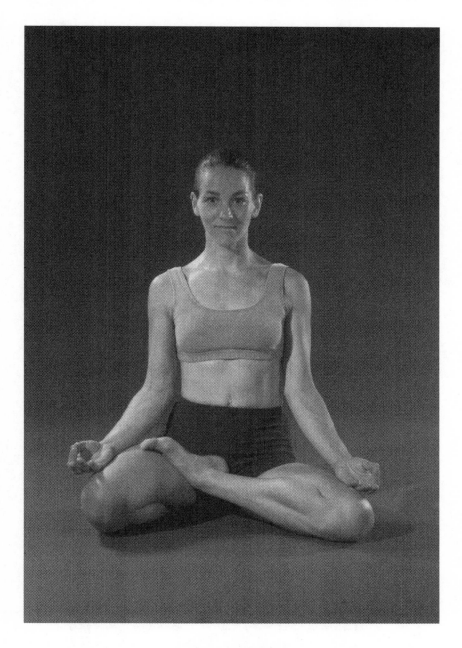

वीरासन – Virasana

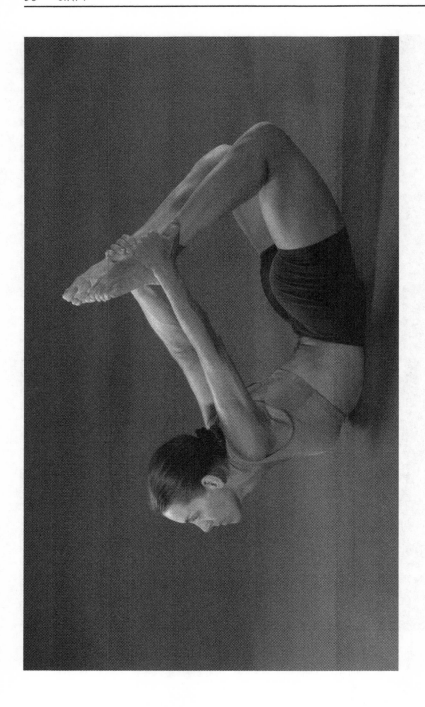

धनुरासन – Dhanurasana

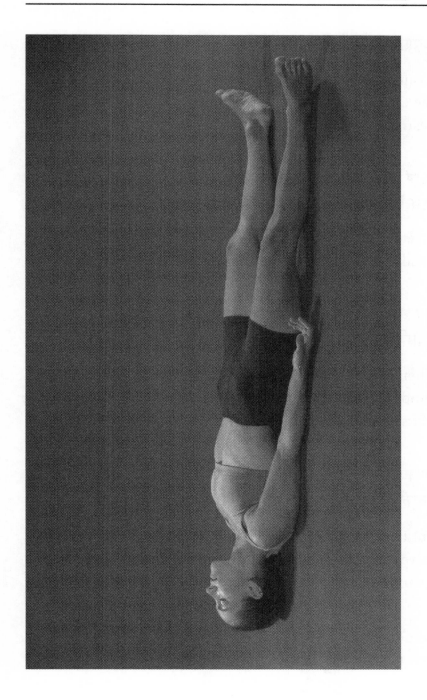

शवासन – Shavasana

कूर्पराभ्यां शिरो वेष्ट्य मत्स्यासनं तु रोगहा ॥ 21

Assume an unbound Padmasana, lie flat out, and wrap
the elbows around the head. This is Matsyasana. It
destroys diseases.

उदरं पश्चिमोत्तानं कृत्वा तिष्ठत्ययत्नतः ।
नमितं वामपदं हि दक्षजानूपरि न्यसेत् ॥ 22

Stretch the abdomen up and backwards without straining,
bend the left leg, and put the left foot on the right knee.

तत्र याम्यं कूर्परं च याम्यकरे च वक्त्रकम् ।
भ्रुवोर्मध्ये गता दृष्टिः पीठं मत्स्येन्द्रमुच्यते ॥ 23

Then put the right elbow there, the face in the right
hand, and the gaze between the eyebrows. This is called
Matsyendrasana.

जानूर्वोरन्तरे पादौ उत्तानौ व्यक्तसंस्थितौ ।
गुल्फौ चाच्छाद्य हस्ताभ्यामुत्तानाभ्यं प्रयत्नतः ॥ 24

Put the feet (turned upwards in plain view) between the
calves and the thighs and carefully cover the heels with
upturned hands.

कण्ठसंकोचनं कृत्वा नासाग्रमवलोकयेत् ।
गोरक्षासनमित्याहुर्योगिनां सिद्धिकारणम् ॥ 25

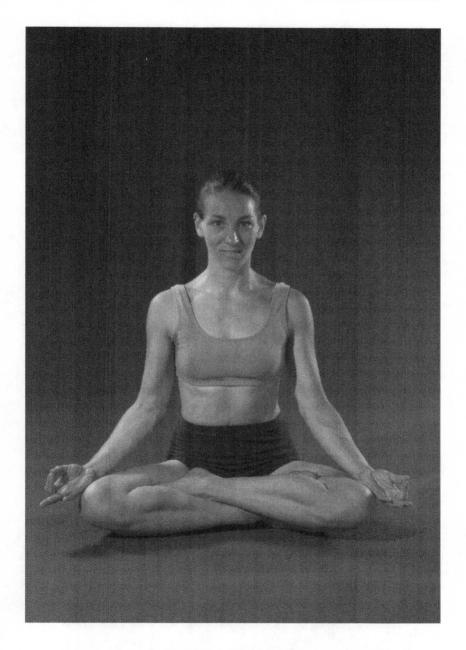

गुप्तासन – Guptasana

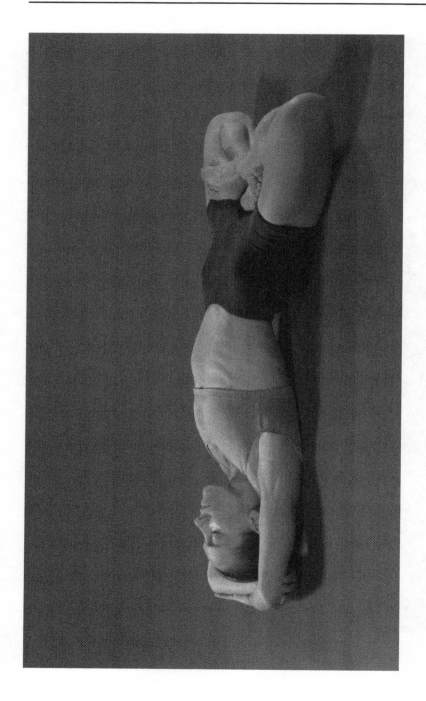

मत्स्यासन – *Matsyasana*

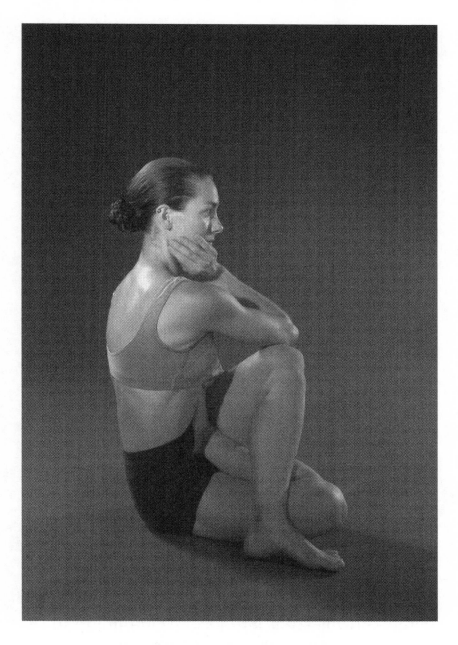

मत्स्येन्द्रासन – Matsyendrasana

Contract the throat and look at the tip of the nose. This is called Gorakshasana. It brings success to yogis.

प्रसार्य पादौ भुवि दण्डरूपौ विन्यस्तभालं चितियुग्ममध्ये ।
यत्नेन पादौ च धृतौ कराभ्यां तत्पश्चिमोत्तानमिहासनं स्यात् ॥ 26

Stretch the legs out on the ground like a stick, put the forehead between the shins, and carefully take hold of the feet with the hands. That is Paschimottanasana.

अङ्गुष्ठाभ्यामवष्टभ्य धरां गुल्फौ च खे गतौ ।
तत्रोपरि गुदं न्यसेद्द्विज्ञेयमुत्कटासनम् ॥ 27

Put the big toes on the ground (taking the weight), the ankles in the air, and the anus on the ankles. This is known as Utkatasana.

वामपादर्चितेर्मूलं विन्यस्य धरणीतले ।
पाददण्डेन याम्येन वेष्टयेद्वामपादकम् ।
जानुयुग्मे करयुग्ममेतत्संकटमासनम् ॥ 28

Put the left shin on the ground, wrap the right leg around the left, and put the hands on the knees. This is Sankatasana.

पाण्योस्तलाभ्यामवलम्ब्य भूमिं तत्कूर्परस्थापितनाभिपार्श्वम् ।
उच्चासनो दण्डवदुत्थितः खे मयूरमेतत्प्रवदन्ति पीठम् ॥ 29

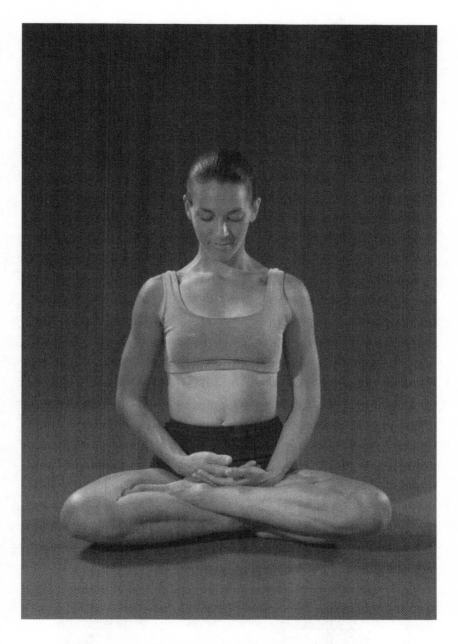

गोरक्षासन – Gorakshasana

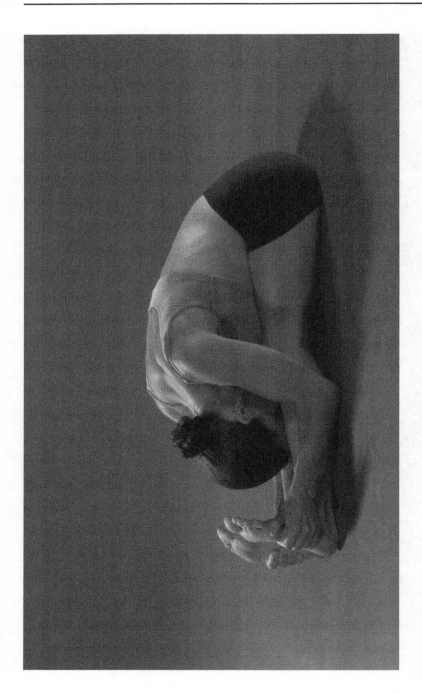

पश्चिमोत्तानासन – Paschimottanasana

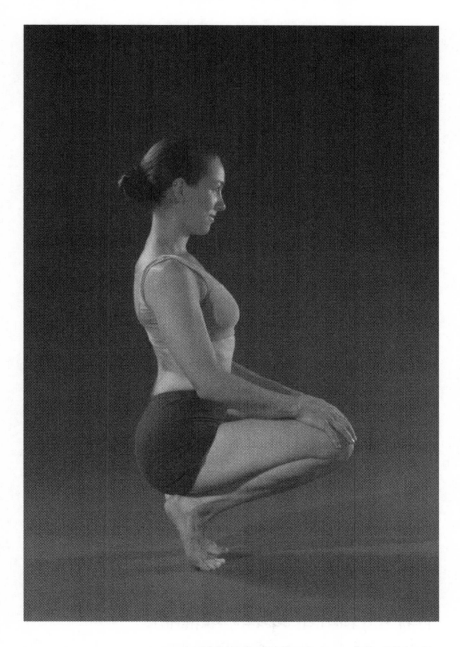

उत्कटासन – Utkatasana

Support yourself with the palms of both hands on the ground, place the elbows on either side of the navel, and raise yourself into the air like a stick. This is called Mayurasana.

बहु कदशनभुक्तं भस्म कुर्यादशेषं
जनयति जठराग्निं जारयेत्कालकूटम् ।
हरति सकलरोगानाशु गुल्मज्वरादीन्
भवति विगतदोषं ह्यासनं श्रीमयूरम् ॥ ३०

The glorious Mayurasana turns to ash all excess, unwholesome food that has been eaten, increases the gastric fire, digests lethal poison, quickly overcomes all diseases such as intestinal tumors, fever, and so forth, and has no disadvantages.

पद्मासनं समासाद्य जानूर्वोरन्तरे करौ ।
कूर्पराभ्यां समासीनो उच्चस्थः कुक्कुटासनम् ॥ ३१

Sit in Padmasana, put the hands between the calves and the thighs, and raise yourself up to the elbows. This is Kukkutasana.

गुल्फौ च वृषणस्याधो व्युत्क्रमेण समाहितौ ।
ऋजुकायशिरोग्रीवं कूर्मासनमितीरितम् ॥ ३२

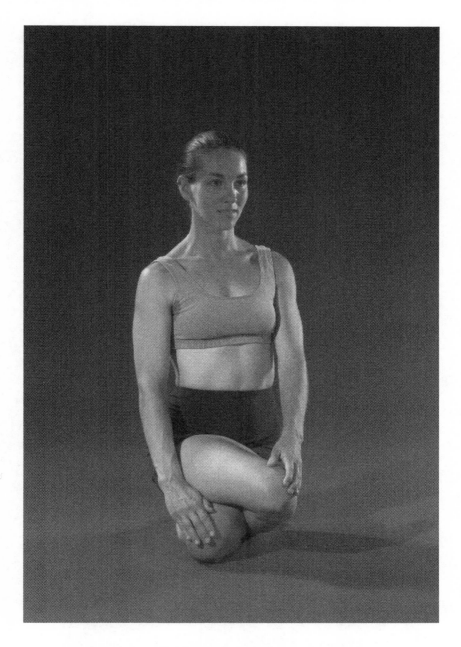

संकटासन – Sankatasana

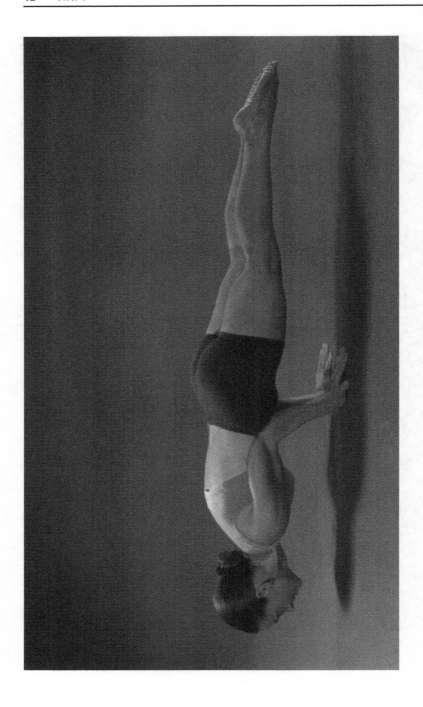

मयूरासन – Mayurasana

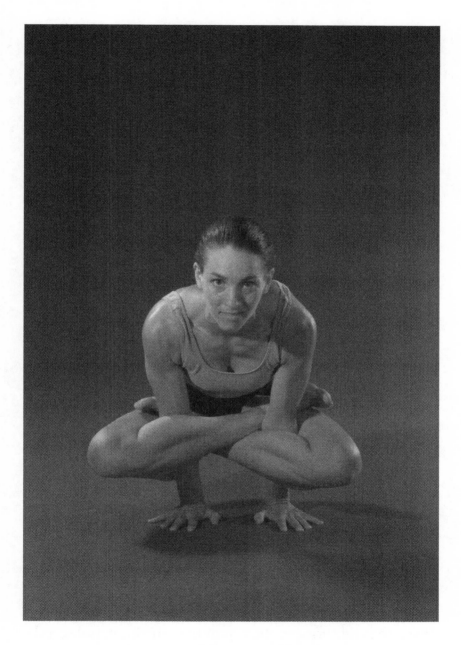

कुक्कुटासन – Kukkutasana

Put both heels together, turn them back below the scrotum, and keep the body, head, and neck straight. This is Kurmasana.

कुक्कुटासनबन्धस्थं कराभ्यां धृतकन्धरम् ।
पीठं कूर्मवदुत्तानमेतदुत्तानकूर्मकम् ॥ ३३

Hold the neck with both hands while in Kukkutasana: this asana, which is like a tortoise on its back, is Uttanakurmakasana.

पृष्ठदेशे पादतलावङ्गुष्ठौ द्वौ च संस्पृशेत् ।
जानुयुग्मं पुरस्कृत्य साधयेन्मण्डुकासनम् ॥ ३४

By putting the soles of both feet in the region of the bottom, touching the big toes together, and keeping the knees in front, the yogi accomplishes Mandukasana.

मण्डुकासनबन्धस्थं कूर्पराभ्यां धृतं शिरः ।
एतद्भेकवदुत्तानमेतदुत्तानमण्डुकम् ॥ ३५

While in Mandukasana, hold the head with the elbows. This, resembling an upright frog, is Uttanamandukasana.

वामोरुमूलदेशे च याम्यं पादं निधाय वै ।
तिष्ठेत्तु वृक्षवद्भूमौ वृक्षासनमिदं विदुः ॥ ३६

Place the right foot at the top of the left thigh and stand on the ground like a tree. This is called Vrikshasana.

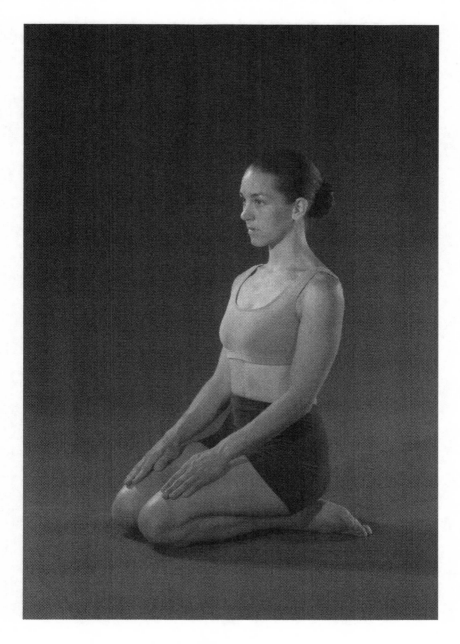

कूर्मासन – Kurmasana

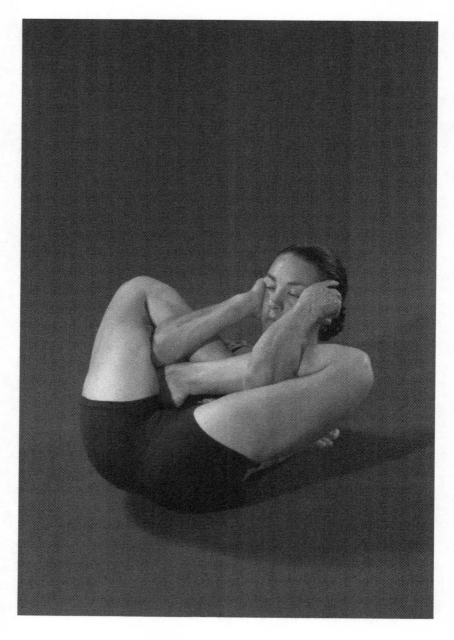

उत्तानकूर्मासन – Uttanakurmasana

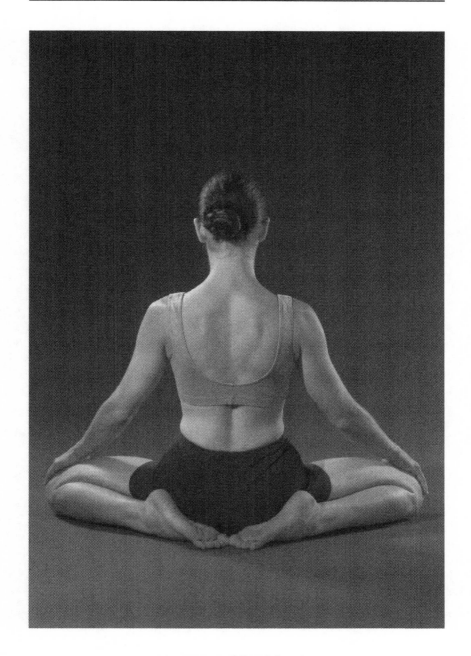

मण्डुकासन – Mandukasana

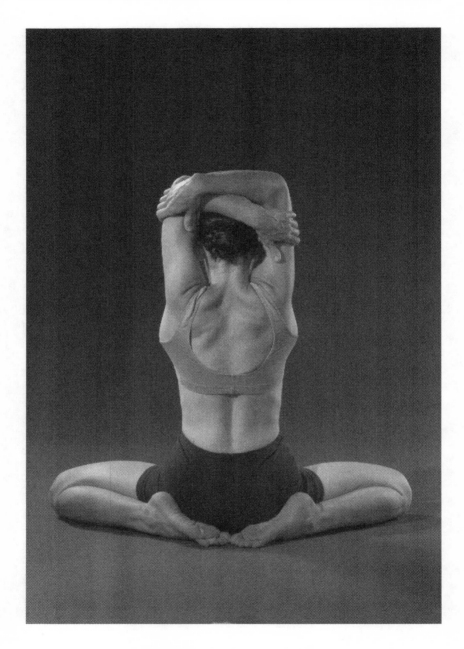

उत्तानमण्डुकासन – Uttanamandukasana

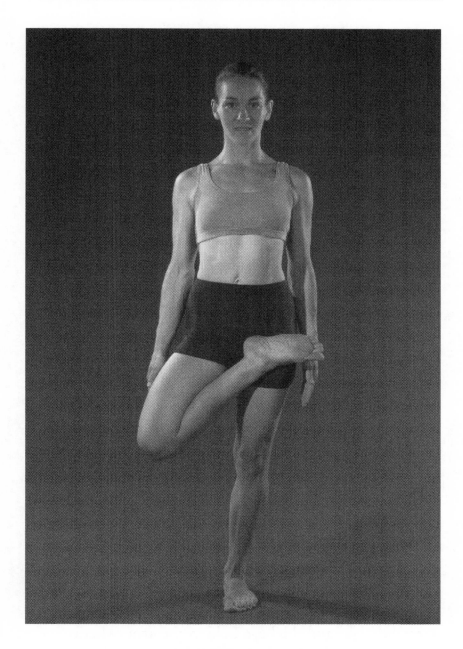

वृक्षासन – Vrikshasana

जङ्घोरुभ्यां धरां पीड्य स्थिरकायो द्विजानुना ।
जानूपरि करद्वन्द्वं गरुडासनमुच्यते ॥ 37

Press both the thighs and the shins against the ground
by means of the two knees, hold the body steady, and put
both hands on the knees. This is called Garudasana.

याम्यगुल्फे पायुमूलं वामभागे पदेतरम् ।
विपरीतं स्पृशेद्भूमिं वृषासनमिदं भवेत् ॥ 38

With the anus on the right ankle, on the left side the
other foot should be turned back and touching the
ground. This is Vrishasana.

अध्यास्य शेते करयुग्मवक्ष आलम्ब्य भूमिं करयोस्तलाभ्याम् ।
पादौ च शून्ये च वितस्ति चोर्ध्वं वदन्ति पीठं शलभं मुनीन्द्राः ॥ 39

Lie prone with the hands by the chest, rest both palms
on the ground, and raise the feet nine inches into the air.
The master sages call this Shalabhasana.

अध्यास्य शेते हृदयं निधाय भूमौ च पादौ प्रविसार्यमाणौ ।
शिरश्च धृत्वा करदण्डयुग्मे देहाग्निकारं मकरासनं तत् ॥ 40

Lie down with the chest placed on the ground, the legs
stretched out, and the head held in the arms: that is
Makarasana. It stokes the bodily fire.

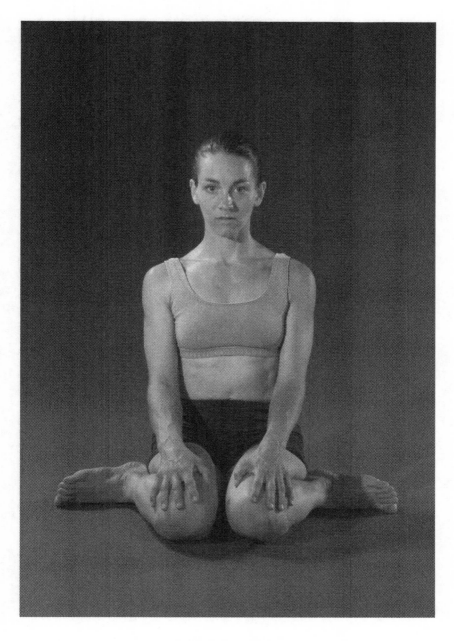

गरुडासन – Garudasana

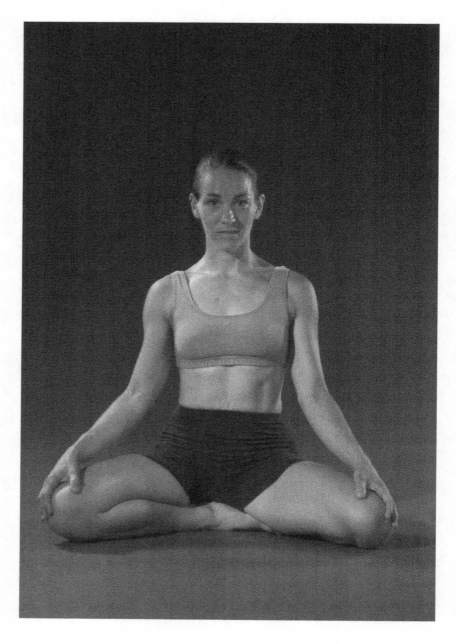

वृषासन – Vrishasana

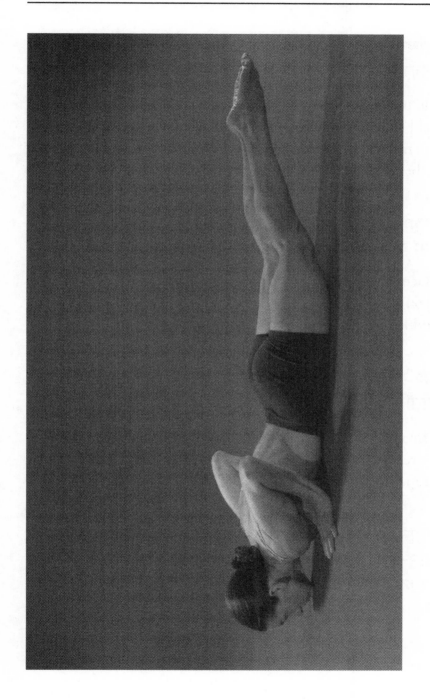

शलभासन – Shalabhasana

अध्यास्य शेते पदयुग्मव्यस्तं पृष्ठे निधायापि धृतं कराभ्याम् ।
आकुञ्च्य सम्यग्घ्युदरास्यगाढमौष्ट्रं च पीठं यतयो वदन्ति ॥ 41

Lie prone with both legs crossed, placed on the back, and held in the hands, and firmly draw in the abdomen and the mouth at the same time. The sages call this Ushtrasana.

अङ्गुष्ठनाभिपर्यन्तमधो भूमौ च विन्यसेत् ।
धरां करतलाभ्यां धृत्वोर्ध्वशीर्षः फणीव हि ॥ 42

Place the lower body, from the toes to the navel, on the ground. Support yourself with both palms on the ground and lift up the head like a snake.

देहाग्निर्वर्धते नित्यं सर्वरोगविनाशनम् ।
जागर्ति भुजगी देवी भुजङ्गासनसाधनात् ॥ 43

Through practice of Bhujangasana, the physical fire increases steadily, all diseases are destroyed, and the Serpent Goddess awakens.

उत्तानौ चरणौ कृत्वा संस्थाप्योपरि जानुनोः ।
आसनोपरि संस्थाप्य चोत्तानं करयुग्मकम् ॥ 44
पूरकैर्वायुमाकृष्य नासाग्रमवलोकयेत् ।
योगासनं भवेदेतद्योगिनां योगसाधनम् ॥ 45

Turn the feet upwards, put them on the knees, place the upturned hands on the ground, inhale repeatedly to draw

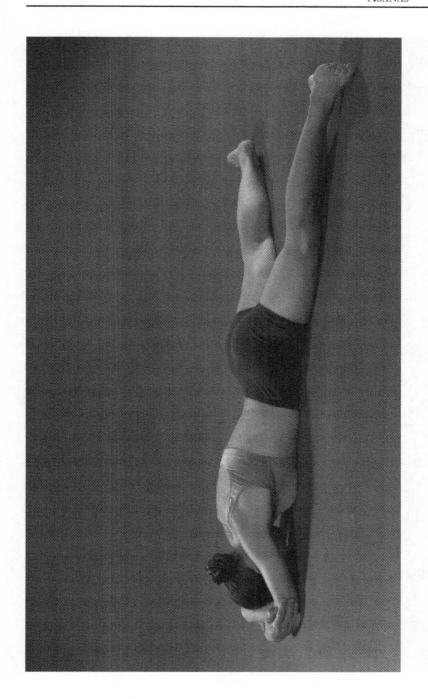

मकरासन – Makarasana

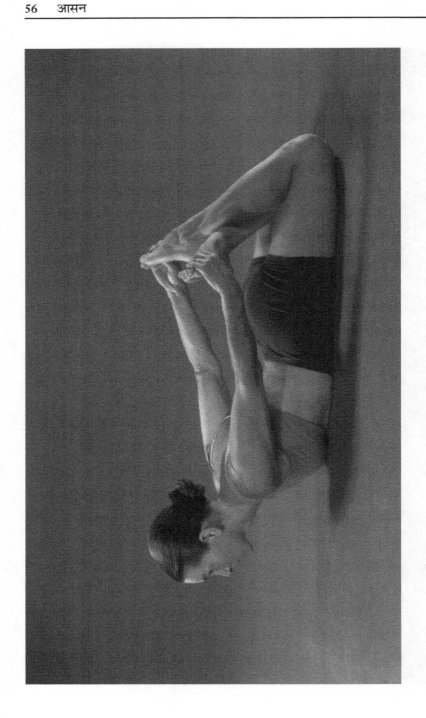

उष्ट्रासन – Ushtrasana

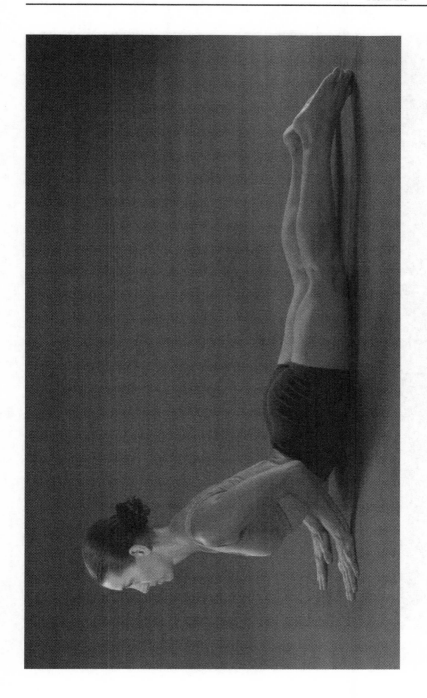

भुजंगासन – Bhujangasana

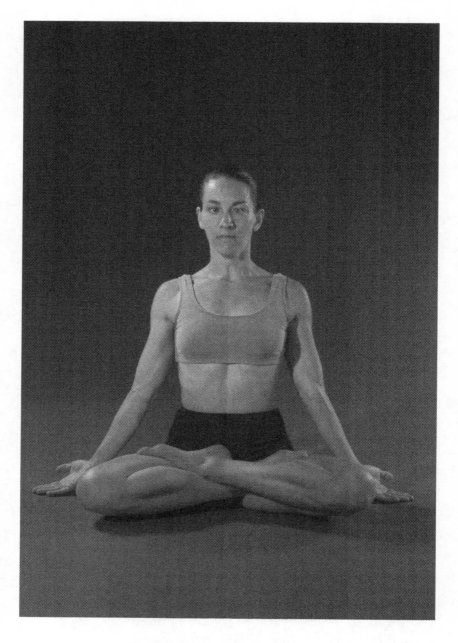

योगासन – Yogasana

in air, and look at the tip of the nose. This is Yogasana, the means for yogis to succeed in Yoga.

इति श्रीघेरण्डसंहितायां घेरण्डचण्डसंवादे
घटस्थयोग आसनप्रयोगो नाम द्वितीयोपदेशः ॥

Thus ends the second chapter, called the practice of asana, in the glorious Gheranda Samhita, a dialogue between Gheranda and Chanda on bodily Yoga.

तृतीयोपदेशः
Chapter Three

Mudras

महामुद्रा नभोमुद्रा उड्डीयानं जलन्धरम् ।
मूलबन्धो महाबन्धो महावेधश्च खेचरी ॥ 1
विपरीतकरी योनिर्वज्रोली शक्तिचालनी ।
ताडागी माण्डुकीमुद्रा शाम्भवी पञ्चधारणा ॥ 2
अश्विनी पाशिनी काकी मातङ्गी च भुजंगिनी ।
पञ्चविंशतिमुद्राश्च सिद्धिदा इह योगिनाम् ॥ 3

Mahamudra, Nabhomudra, Uddiyana, Jalandhara,
Mulabandha, Mahabandha, Mahavedha, and Khechari;
Viparitakarani, Yoni, Vajroli, Shaktichalani, Tadagi,
Mandukimudra, Shambhavi, the five dharanas, Ashvini,
Pashini, Kaki, Matangi, and Bhujangini: these twenty-five
mudras grant success in this world to yogis.

पायुमूलं वामगुल्फे संपीड्य दृढयत्नतः ।
याम्यपादं प्रसार्याथ करोपात्तपदाङ्गुलिः ॥ 4
कण्ठसंकोचनं कृत्वा भ्रुवोर्मध्ये निरीक्षयेत् ।
पूरकैर्वायुं संपूर्य महामुद्रा निगद्यते ॥ 5

Firmly press the anus onto the left ankle, extend the right foot, hold the toes with the hands, contract the throat, and look between the eyebrows. Inhaling repeatedly, fill yourself completely with air. This is called Mahamudra.

वलितं पलितं चैव जरामृत्युं निवारयेत् ।
क्षयकासगुदावर्तप्लीहाजीर्णज्वरं तथा ।
नाशयेत्सर्वरोगांश्च महामुद्राप्रसाधनात् ॥ ६

It can cure wrinkles and gray hair, old age and death, consumptive cough, constipation, disorders of the spleen, decrepitude, and fever. By mastering Mahamudra, the yogi can get rid of all diseases.

यत्र यत्र स्थितो योगी सर्वकार्येषु सर्वदा ।
ऊर्ध्वजिह्नः स्थिरो भूत्वा धारयेत्पवनं सदा ।
नभोमुद्रा भवेदेषा योगिनां रोगनाशिनी ॥ ७

Wherever the yogi may be, he should always, in everything he does, be sure to keep the tongue turned upwards and constantly hold the breath. This is Nabhomudra, the destroyer of diseases for yogis.

उदरे पश्चिमं तानं नाभेरूर्ध्वं तु कारयेत् ।
उड्डीनं कुरुते यस्मादविश्रान्तं महाखगः ।
उड्डीयानं त्वसौ बन्धो मृत्युमातंगकेसरी ॥ ८

Draw the abdomen backwards above the navel so that the great bird flies unceasingly upwards. This is Uddiyana-bandha, a lion against the elephant of death.

समग्राद्बन्धनाद्ध्येतदुड्डीयानं विशिष्यते ।
उड्डीयाने समभ्यस्ते मुक्तिः स्वाभाविकी भवेत् ॥ ९

This Uddiyana sets itself apart from all bandhas: when Uddiyana is practiced, liberation arises spontaneously.

कण्ठसंकोचनं कृत्वा चिबुकं हृदये न्यसेत् ।
जालन्धरे कृते बन्धे षोडशाधारबन्धनम् ।
जालन्धरमहामुद्रा मृत्योश्च क्षयकारिणी ॥ १०

Contract the throat and put the chin on the chest. When Jalandharabandha is performed, the sixteen adharas are restrained.[1] The great Jalandhara mudra brings about death's downfall.

सिद्धो जालन्धरो बन्धो योगिनां सिद्धिदायकः ।
षण्मासमभ्यसेद्यो हि स सिद्धो नात्र संशयः ॥ ११

A perfected Jalandharabandha bestows success upon yogis. He who practices it for six months is an adept. In this there is no doubt.

---

[1] A bandha (lock) is a type of mudra. The sixteen adharas (literally "supports" or "substrates") are at various locations within the body. They are listed in the *Siddha Siddhanta Paddhati*, verses 2.10–25.

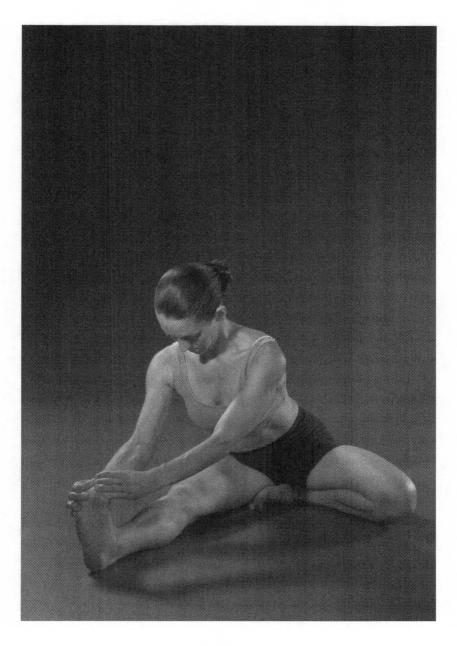

महामुद्रा – Mahamudra

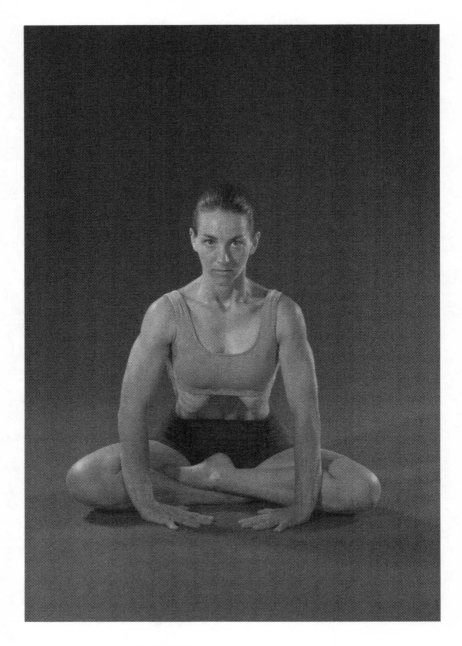

उड्डीयानबन्ध – Uddiyanabandha

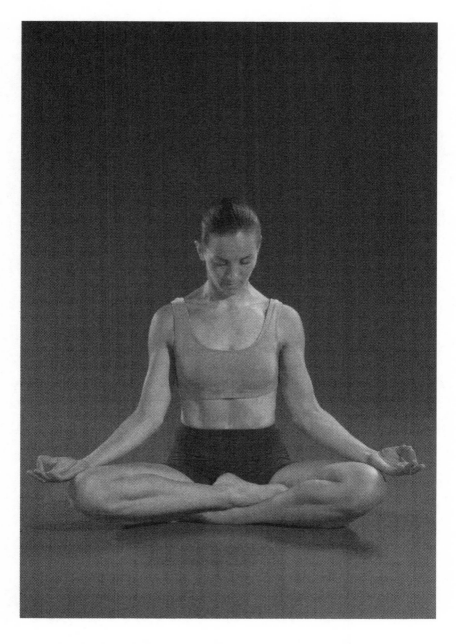

जालन्धरबन्ध & मूलबन्ध – Jalandharabandha & Mulabandha

पार्ष्णिना वामपादस्य योनिमाकुञ्चयेत्ततः ।
नाभिग्रन्थिं मेरुदण्डे सुधीः संपीड्य यत्नतः ॥ 12

The wise yogi should apply pressure to the perineum
with the heel of the left foot and carefully push the navel
plexus against the spine.

मेढ्रं दक्षिणगुल्केन दृढबन्धं समाचरेत् ।
जराविनाशिनी मुद्रा मूलबन्धो निगद्यते ॥ 13

He should tightly press the penis with the right heel. This
mudra destroys decrepitude and is called Mulabandha.

वामपादस्य गुल्केन पायुमूलं निरोधयेत् ।
दक्षपादेन तद्गुल्कं संपीड्य यत्नतः सुधीः ॥ 14

With the ankle of his left foot the wise yogi should block
the anus, and with the right foot he should carefully press
down on the left ankle.

शनकैश्चालयेत्पार्ष्णिं योनिमाकुञ्चयेच्छनैः ।
जालन्धरे धारयेत्प्राणं महाबन्धो निगद्यते ॥ 15

He should slowly move his heel about, gently contract the
perineum, and hold the breath in Jalandharabandha. This
is called Mahabandha.

महाबन्धः परो बन्धो जरामरणनाशनः ।

प्रसादादस्य बन्धस्य साधयेत्सर्ववाञ्छितम् ॥ 16

Mahabandha is a great bandha: it destroys decrepitude and death, and by its grace the yogi can achieve whatever he wants.

रूपयौवनलावण्यं नारीणां पुरुषं विना ।
मूलबन्धमहाबन्धौ महावेधं विना तथा ॥ 17

Mulabandha and Mahabandha without Mahavedha are like the beauty, youth, and charm of a woman without a man.

महाबन्धं समासाद्य चरेदुड्डानकुम्भकं ।
महावेधः समाख्यातो योगिनां सिद्धिदायकः ॥ 18

Assume Mahabandha and hold the breath while applying Uddiyanabandha. This is called Mahavedha. It bestows success upon yogis.

महाबन्धमूलबन्धौ महावेधसमन्वितौ ।
प्रत्यहं कुरुते यस्तु स योगी योगवित्तमः ॥ 19

The yogi who every day practices Mahabandha and Mulabandha combined with Mahavedha is the best of Yoga experts.

न मृत्युतो भयं तस्य न जरा तस्य विद्यते ।
गोपनीयः प्रयत्नेन वेधोऽयं योगिपुंगवैः ॥ 20

He has no fear of death and does not become decrepit. This
Mahavedha is to be kept secret by the masters of Yoga.

जिह्वाधोनाडीं संछित्य रसनां चालयेत्सदा ।
दोहयेन्नवनीतेन लौहयन्त्रेण कर्षयेत् ॥ 21

The yogi should regularly cut the tendon below the
tongue and move the tongue about. He should milk it
with fresh butter and pull it with iron tongs.

एवं नित्यं समभ्यासाल्लम्बिका दीर्घतां व्रजेत् ।
यावन्नच्छेद्भ्रुवोर्मध्ये तदा सिध्यति खेचरी ॥ 22

By regular practice in this way, the tongue becomes long.
When it reaches between the eyebrows, Khechari
is perfected.

रसनां तालुमूले तु शनैः शनैः प्रवेशयेत् ।
कपालकुहरे जिह्वा प्रविष्टा विपरीतगा ।
भ्रुवोर्मध्ये गता दृष्टिर्मुद्रा भवति खेचरी ॥ 23

Gently insert the tongue into the base of the palate.
When the tongue is turned back into the cavity of the
skull and the gaze is directed between the eyebrows, that
is Khecharimudra.

न च मूर्च्छा क्षुधा तृष्णा नैवालस्यं प्रजायते ।
न च रोगो जरा मृत्युर्देवदेहः स जायते ॥ 24

Loss of consciousness, hunger, thirst, sloth, sickness, decrepitude, and death do not arise, and the yogi obtains the body of a god.

न चाग्निर्दहते गात्रं न शोषयति मारुतः ।
न देहं क्लेदयन्त्यापो दशेन्न च भुजङ्गमः ॥ 25

Fire does not burn the body, the winds do not dry it out, water does not wet it, and a snake cannot bite it.

लावण्यं च भवेद्गात्रे समाधिर्जायते ध्रुवम् ।
कपालवक्त्रसंयोगे रसना रसमाप्नुयात् ॥ 26

The body becomes beautiful and samadhi is sure to arise. When it comes into contact with the aperture of the skull, the tongue reaches a liquid.

नानारससमुद्भूतमानन्दं च दिने दिने ।
आदौ च लवणं क्षारं ततस्तिक्तकषायकम् ॥ 27
नवनीतं घृतं क्षीरं दधितक्रमधूनि च ।
द्राक्षारसं च पीयूषं जायते रसनोदकम् ॥ 28

Each day a blissful sensation arises from the various flavors. At first the fluid on the tongue is salty and brackish, then bitter and sharp, then like fresh butter, ghee, milk, curd, buttermilk, honey, grape juice, and nectar.

नाभिमूले वसेत्सूर्यस्तालुमूले च चन्द्रमाः ।

अमृतं ग्रसते सूर्यस्ततो मृत्युवशो नरः ॥ 29

The sun dwells at the root of the navel, and the moon at the root of the palate. The sun consumes the nectar of immortality and thus man is held in the sway of death.

ऊर्ध्वं च योजयेत्सूर्यं चन्द्रं चाप्यध आनयेत् ।
विपरीतकरी मुद्रा सर्वतन्त्रेषु गोपिता ॥ 30

Put the sun up and bring the moon down. This Viparita-karani mudra is concealed in all the tantras.

भूमौ शिरश्च संस्थाप्य करयुग्मं समाहितः ।
ऊर्ध्वपादः स्थिरो भूत्वा विपरीतकरी मता ॥ 31

Carefully place the head and both hands on the ground, raise the feet, and remain steady. This is considered to be Viparitakarani.

मुद्रां च साधयेन्नित्यं जरां मृत्युं च नाशयेत् ।
स सिद्धः सर्वलोकेषु प्रलयेऽपि न सीदति ॥ 32

He who regularly practices this mudra destroys decrepitude and death, is an adept in all the worlds, and does not perish even at the great dissolution.

सिद्धासनं समासाद्य कर्णचक्षुर्नसामुखम् ।
अङ्गुष्ठतर्जनीमध्यानामादौः पिदधीत वै ॥ 33

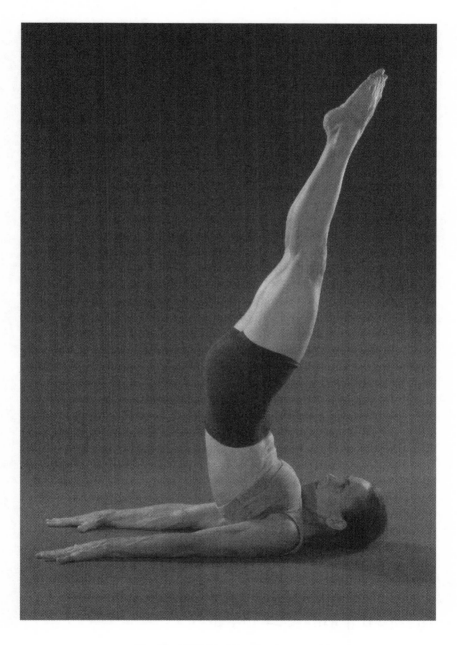

विपरीतकरणी – Viparitakarani

The yogi should sit in Siddhasana and block the ears with the thumbs, the eyes with the index fingers, the nostrils with the middle fingers, and the mouth with the ring and little fingers.

प्राणमाकृष्य काकीभिरपाने योजयेत्ततः ।
षट्चक्राणि क्रमाद्धयात्वा हुंहंसमनुना सुधीः ॥ ३४
चैतन्यमानयेद्देवीं निद्रिता या भुजंगिनी ।
जीवेन सहितां शक्तिं समुत्थाप्य पराम्बुजे ॥ ३५

Having drawn in prana with repeated applications of Kakimudra, he should then join it with apana and meditate on the six chakras in succession. Using the mantras *hum* and *hamsa*, the wise yogi should bring the sleeping Serpent Goddess to consciousness and raise her, together with the jiva, to the highest lotus.

स्वयं शक्तिमयो भूत्वा परं शिवेन संगमम् ।
नानासुखं विहारं च चिन्तयेत्परमं सुखम् ॥ ३६

Having himself now become made of Shakti, he should visualize supreme union with Shiva, as well as various pleasures, enjoyments, and ultimate bliss.

शिवशक्तिसमायोगादेकान्तं भुवि भावयेत् ।
आनन्दमानसो भूत्वा अहं ब्रह्मेति संभवेत् ॥ ३७

As a result of the union of Shiva and Shakti, he should experience the ultimate goal on earth. With blissful mind, he should realize that he is Brahman.

योनिमुद्रा परा गोप्या देवानामपि दुर्लभा ।
सकृत्तु लब्धसंसिद्धिः समाधिस्थः स एव हि ॥ 38

The great Yonimudra is to be kept secret. It is hard to obtain even for the gods. As soon as he masters it the yogi is sure to enter samadhi.

आश्रित्य भूमिं करयोस्तलाभ्यामूर्ध्वं क्षिपेत्पादयुगं शिरः खे ।
शक्तिप्रबुद्ध्यै चिरजीवनाय वज्रोलिमुद्रां मुनयो वदन्ति ॥ 39

Support yourself on the ground with the palms of both hands and raise the head and feet into the air. The sages prescribe this Vajrolimudra to awaken Shakti and bring about a long life.

मूलाधारे आत्मशक्तिः कुण्डली परदेवता ।
शयिता भुजगाकारा सार्धत्रिवलयान्विता ॥ 40

The great goddess Kundalini, the Shakti of the self, sleeps at the Muladhara in the form of a snake with three and one-half coils.

यावत्सा निद्रिता देहे तावज्जीवः पशुर्यथा ।
ज्ञानं न जायते तावत्कोटियोगं समभ्यसेत् ॥ 41

As long as she is asleep in the body, the jiva is but a bound animal and gnosis does not arise, even if the yogi practices innumerable Yogas.

उद्घाटयेत्कवाटं च यथा कुञ्चिकया हठात् ।
कुण्डलिन्याः प्रबोधेन ब्रह्मद्वारं प्रभेदयेत् ॥ 42

Just as he might open a door with a key, so should the yogi forcefully awaken Kundalini and break open the gateway of Brahman.

नाभिं संवेष्ट्य वस्त्रेण न च नग्नं बहिः स्थितम् ।
गोपनीयगृहे स्थित्वा शक्तिचालनमभ्यसेत् ॥ 43

Wrap the midriff in a cloth, don't go outside while naked, and stay in a private room to practice Shaktichalana.

वितस्तिप्रमितं दीर्घं विस्तारे चतुरङ्गुलम् ।
मृदुलं धवलं सूक्ष्मं वेष्टनाम्बरलक्षणम् ।
एवमम्बरयुक्तं च कटिसूत्रेण योजयेत् ॥ 44

The covering cloth should be nine inches long, three inches wide, soft, white, and fine. Put on such a covering and tie it to the string around the waist.

संलिप्य भास्मना गात्रं सिद्धासनमथाचरेत् ।
नासाभ्यां प्राणमाकृष्याप्यपाने योजयेद्बलात् ॥ 45

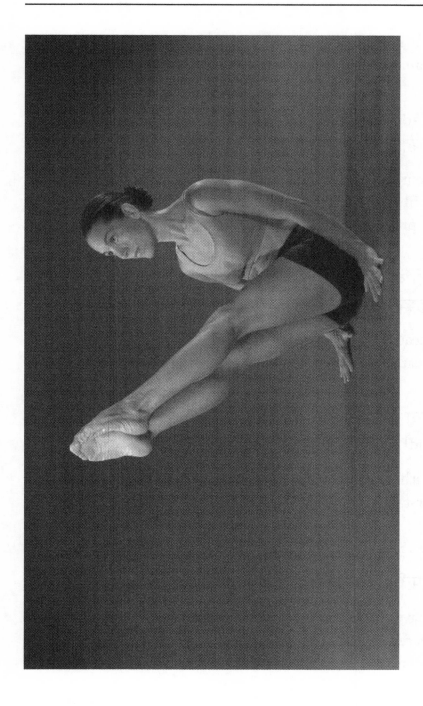

वज्रोलिमुद्रा – Vajrolimudra

Smear the body with ash and sit in Siddhasana. Draw in prana through the nostrils and force it to join with apana.

तावदाकुञ्चयेत्तुह्यमश्विनीमुद्रया शनैः ।
यावन्नच्छेत्सुषुम्णायां हठाद्वायुः प्रकाशयेत् ॥ ४६

Gently contract the anus by means of Ashvinimudra until air is forced to enter the Sushumna and manifest its presence.

तदा वायुप्रबन्धेन कुम्भिका च भुजंगिनी ।
बद्धश्वासस्ततो भूत्वा चोर्ध्वमार्गं प्रपद्यते ॥ ४७

Because the air has been restricted, Kundalini holds her breath and suffocates, then enters the upward path.

विना शक्तिचालनेन योनिमुद्रा न सिध्यति ।
आदौ चालनमभ्यस्य योनिमुद्रां ततोऽभ्यसेत् ॥ ४८

Without Shaktichalana, Yonimudra does not succeed. First practice Shaktichalana and then practice Yonimudra.

इति ते कथितं चण्डकपाले शक्तिचालनम् ।
गोपनीयं प्रयत्नेन दिने दिने समभ्यसेत् ॥ ४९

I have thus taught you Shaktichalana, Chanda the Skull-bearer. It should be carefully kept secret and practiced every day.

उदरं पश्चिमोत्तानं तडागाकृति कारयेत् ।
तडागी सा परा मुद्रा जरामृत्युविनाशिनी ॥ 50

Draw the belly backwards and upwards so that it looks
like a pond. This is the great Tadagimudra. It destroys
decrepitude and death.

मुखं संमुद्रितं कृत्वा जिह्वामूलं प्रचालयेत् ।
शनैर्ग्रसेत्तदमृतं माण्डुकीं मुद्रिकां विदुः ॥ 51

Seal the mouth and move the base of the tongue about.
Then slowly swallow the nectar of immortality. This is
called Mandukimudra.

वलितं पलितं नैव जायते नित्ययौवनम् ।
न केशे जायते पाको यः कुर्यान्नित्यमाण्डुकीम् ॥ 52

For the man who regularly practices Manduki, neither
wrinkles nor old age arise; he gets eternal youth and his
hair does not turn gray.

नेत्रान्तरं समालोक्य चात्मारामं निरीक्षयेत् ।
सा भवेच्छांभवी मुद्रा सर्वतन्त्रेषु गोपिता ॥ 53

Look between the eyes and observe the delights of the
self. This is Shambhavimudra, which is concealed in
all the tantras.

वेदशास्त्रपुराणानि सामान्यगणिका इव ।
इयं तु शाम्भवी मुद्रा गुप्ता कुलवधूरिव ॥ 54

The Vedas, Shastras, and Puranas are like common cour-
tesans; this Shambhavimudra is kept hidden like a lady of
good family.

स एव ह्यादिनाथश्च स च नारायणः स्वयम् ।
स च ब्रह्मा सृष्टिकारी यो मुद्रां वेत्ति शाम्भवीम् ॥ 55

He who knows Shambhavimudra is none other than Adi-
natha, he is Narayana himself, he is Brahma the Creator.[2]

सत्यं सत्यं पुनः सत्यं सत्यमाह महेश्वर ।
शाम्भवीं यो विजानीयात्स च ब्रह्म न चान्यथा ॥ 56

Maheshvara has said, 'Truly, truly, and again truly, he
who knows Shambhavi is Brahman—and no one else.'

कथिता शाम्भवी मुद्रा शृणुष्व पञ्चधारणाम् ।
धारणानि समासाद्य किं न सिध्यति भूतले ॥ 57

I have taught you Shambhavimudra. Now hear the five
dharanas. By practicing the dharanas, everything on
earth is possible.

अनेन नरदेहेन स्वर्गेषु गमनागमम् ।

---

[2]Adinatha and Narayana are names of Shiva and Vishnu respectively.

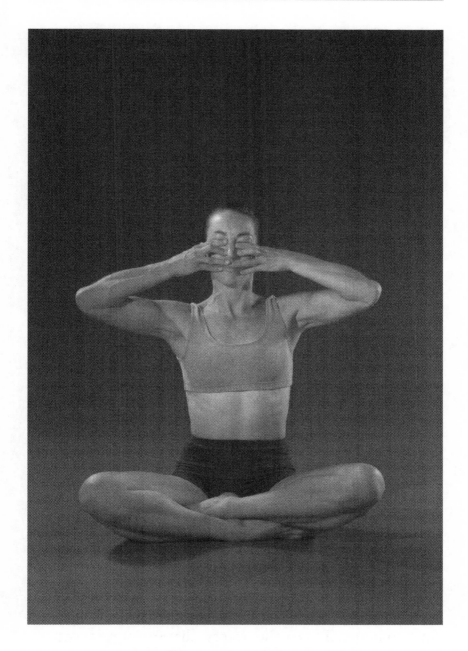

शाम्भवीमुद्रा – Shambhavimudra

मनोगतिर्भवित्तस्य खेचरत्वं न चान्यथा ॥ ५८

The yogi can come and go from the heavenly realms in
his mortal body; he can move as fast as the mind and has
the power of traveling through space. There is no other
way of achieving this.

यत्तत्त्वं हरितालदेशरुचिरं भौमं लकारान्वितं
संयुक्तं कमलासनेन हि चतुष्कोणं हृदि स्थापितम् ।
प्राणं तत्र विलीय पञ्चघटिकाश्चित्तान्वितं धारयेत्
एषा स्तम्भकरी सदा क्षितिजयं कुर्याद्दिवोधारणा ॥ ५९

The earth element shines like a piece of yellow orpiment
and contains the syllable *la*. It is accompanied by Brahma,
is square, and is situated at the heart. Fix the breath and
the mind there for two hours. This is the earthly dharana;
it always brings about steadiness and conquers the earth.

अर्धेन्दुप्रतिमं च कुन्दधवलं कण्ठेऽम्बुतत्त्वं स्थितं
यत्पीयूषवकारबीजसहितं युक्तं सदा विष्णुना ।
प्राणं तत्र विलीय पञ्चघटिकाश्चित्तान्वितं धारयेत्
एषा दुःसहतापपापहरिणी स्यादाम्भसी धारणा ॥ ६०

The water element is situated in the throat. It resembles
a half-moon and is as white as a jasmine flower. It has the
ambrosial syllable *va* as its seed mantra and is always
associated with Vishnu. Fix the breath and the mind there
for two hours. This is the watery dharana. It removes
unbearable suffering and sins.

यत्तालुस्थितमिन्द्रगोपसदृशं तत्त्वं त्रिकोणान्वितं
तेजो रेफमयं प्रदीप्तमरुणं रुद्रेण यत्संगतम् ।
प्राणं तत्र विलीय पञ्चघटिकाश्चित्तान्वितं धारयेद्
एषा कालगभीरभीतिहरणी वैश्वानरी धारणा ॥ 61

The fire element is at the palate. It resembles an Indragopa
insect, consists of a triangle and the syllable *ra*, is blazing
red, and associated with Rudra.[3] Fix the breath and the
mind there for two hours. This fiery dharana removes the
deep fear of death.

यद्बिन्द्वाञ्जनपुञ्जसंनिभमिदं तत्त्वं भुवोरन्तरे
वृत्तं वायुमयं यकारसहितं यत्रेश्वरो देवता ।
प्राणं तत्र विलीय पञ्चघटिकाश्चित्तान्वितं धारयेद्
एषा खे गमनं करोति यमिनां स्याद्वायवी धारणा ॥ 62

The air element is between the eyebrows and looks like
a mass of lampblack. It is a circle, is associated with the
syllable *ya*, and the deity there is Ishvara. Fix the breath
and the mind there for two hours. This airy dharana
brings about the ability to move through space.

आकाशं सुविशुद्धवारिसदृशं यद्ब्रह्मरन्ध्रे स्थितं
तत्राद्येन सदाशिवेन सहितं तत्त्वं हकारान्वितम् ।
प्राणं तत्र विलीय पञ्चघटिकाश्चित्तान्वितं धारयेद्
एषा मोक्षकवाटपाटनपटुः प्रोक्ता नभोधारणा ॥ 63

---

[3]The Indragopa insect, a variety of cochineal, is bright red.

The space element is at the aperture of Brahman and
looks like the clearest water. It is associated there with the
primordial Sadashiva and it contains the syllable *ha*.[4] Fix
the breath and the mind there for two hours. This sky
dharana is said to be able to break down the doorway
to liberation.

आकुञ्चयेन्नुदद्द्वारं प्रकाशयेत्पुनः पुनः ।
सा भवेदश्विनी मुद्रा शक्तिप्रबोधकारिणी ॥ 64

Contract and dilate the anus over and over again. This is
Ashvinimudra. It awakens Shakti.

कण्ठपृष्ठे क्षिपेत्पादौ पाशवद्दृढबन्धनम् ।
सैव स्यात्पाशिनी मुद्रा शक्तिप्रबोधकारिणी ॥ 65

Put the feet behind the neck, making a tight restraint like
a noose. This is Pashinimudra. It awakens Shakti.

काकचञ्चुवदास्येन पिबेद्वायुं शनैः शनैः ।
काकी मुद्रा भवेदेषा सर्वरोगविनाशिनी ॥ 66

Make the mouth like a crow's beak and very slowly draw
in air. This is Kakimudra. It destroys all diseases.

---

[4]No shape is given here for visualizing the space element. In other texts it is
circular and the air element (which in this text is circular—see the preceding
verse) is visualized as a ring of six dots.

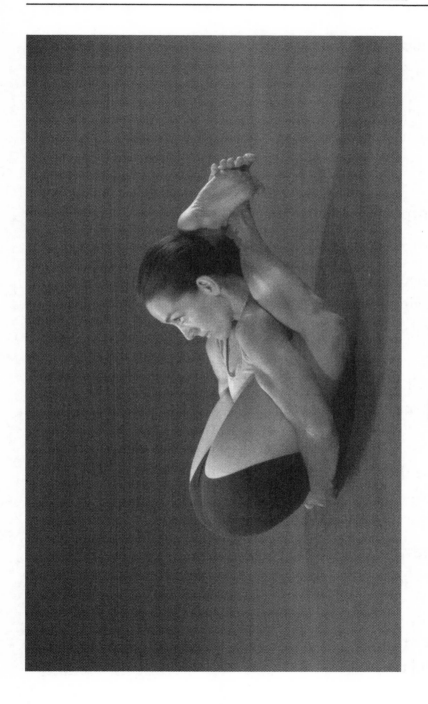

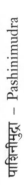

पाशिनीमुद्रा – Pashinimudra

कण्ठदघ्ने जले स्थित्वा नासाभ्यां जलमाहरेत् ।
मुखान्निर्गमयेत्पश्चात्पुनर्वक्त्रेण चाहरेत् ॥ 67

Standing in water up to the neck, draw in water through
the nostrils. Then expel it through the mouth before
drawing it in again through the mouth.

नासाभ्यां रेचयेत्पश्चात्कुर्यदिवं पुनः पुनः ।
मातङ्गिनी परा मुद्रा जरामृत्युविनाशिनी ॥ 68

Then expel it through the nostrils. Do this over and over
again. The great Matangimudra destroys decrepitude
and death.

वक्त्रं किंचित्सुप्रसार्य चानिलं गलया पिबेत् ।
सा भवेद्भुजगी मुद्रा जरामृत्युविनाशिनी ॥ 69

Push the mouth slightly forward and draw in air through
the throat. This is Bhujanginimudra. It destroys decrepitude and death.

यावन्तश्रोदरे रोगा अजीर्णाद्या विशेषतः ।
तान्सर्वान्नाशयेदाशु यत्र मुद्रा भुजंगिनी ॥ 70

The yogi who practices Bhujanginimudra quickly
destroys all gastric ailments, particularly indigestion
and the like.

इति श्रीघेरण्डसंहितायां घेरण्डचण्डसंवादे
घटस्थयोगप्रकरणे मुद्राप्रयोगो नाम तृतीयोपदेशः ॥

Thus ends the third chapter, called the practice of mudra, in the glorious Gheranda Samhita, a dialogue between Gheranda and Chanda and a treatise on bodily Yoga.

चतुर्थोपदेशः

Chapter Four

Pratyahara

अथातः संप्रवक्ष्यामि प्रत्याहारकमुत्तमम् ।
यस्य विज्ञानमात्रेण कामादिरिपुनाशनम् ॥ १

Now I shall teach the sublime pratyahara, the mere understanding of which brings about the destruction of enemies such as passion.

यतो यतो निश्चरति मनश्चञ्चलमस्थिरम् ।
ततस्ततो नियम्यैतदात्मन्येव वशं नयेत् ॥ २

The restless and unsteady mind is to be reined in from wherever it goes and brought under control in the self.

यत्र यत्र गता दृष्टिर्मनस्तत्र प्रयच्छति ।
अतः प्रत्याहरेदेतदात्मन्येव वशं नयेत् ॥ ३

Wherever the sight goes, the mind follows, so draw it back and bring it under control in the self.

पुरस्कारं तिरस्कारं सुश्राव्यं वा भयानकम् ।
मनस्तस्मान्नियम्यैतदात्मन्येव वशं नयेत् ॥ ४

Hold the mind back from sounds, whether compli-
mentary, rude, pleasant, or horrible, and bring it under
control in the self.

शीतं चापि तथा चोष्णं यन्मनःस्पर्शयोगतः ।
तस्मात्प्रत्याहरेदेतदात्मन्येव वशं नयेत् ॥ ५

When the mind comes into contact with something
hot or cold, draw it back from there and bring it under
control in the self.

सुगन्धे वापि दुर्गन्धे मनो घ्राणेषु जायते ।
तस्मात्प्रत्याहरेदेतदात्मन्येव वशं नयेत् ॥ ६

When the mind turns toward smells, good or bad, draw it
back from them and bring it under control in the self.

मधुराम्लकतिक्तादिरसं गतं यदा मनः ।
तस्मात्प्रत्याहरेदेतदात्मन्येव वशं नयेत् ॥ ७

When the mind turns toward tastes, such as sweet, sour,
and bitter, draw it back from them and bring it under
control in the self.

इति श्रीघेरण्डसंहितायां घेरण्डचण्डसंवादे घटस्थयोगे

प्रत्याहारप्रयोगो नाम चतुर्थोपदेशः ॥

Thus ends the fourth chapter, called the practice of pratyahara, in the glorious Gheranda Samhita, a dialogue
between Gheranda and Chanda on bodily Yoga.

Pranayama

अथातः संप्रवक्ष्यामि प्राणायामस्य सद्विधिम् ।
यस्य साधनमात्रेण देवतुल्यो भवेन्नरः ॥ 1

Now I shall teach the correct way to practice pranayama,
simply by mastering which a man can become equal
to a god.

आदौ स्थानं तथा कालं मिताहारं तथापरम् ।
नाडीशुद्धिं ततः पश्चात्प्राणायामं च साधयेत् ॥ 2

Before practicing pranayama, first concern yourself with
location and season, then with moderating the diet, and
then with cleansing the nadis.

दूरदेशे तथारण्ये राजधान्यां जनान्तिके ।
योगारम्भं न कुर्वीत कृतश्चेत्सिद्धिहा भवेत् ॥ 3

One should not start a Yoga practice in a remote area, a
forest, a city, or near people. When undertaken in such
places, Yoga is not successful.

अविश्वासं दूरदेशे अरण्ये भक्षवर्जितम् ।
लोकमध्ये प्रकाशश्च तस्मात्रीणि विवर्जयेत् ॥ 4

In a remote area there is no security, in a forest there
is no food, and amongst people there is the glare of
publicity, so avoid these three.

सुदेशे धार्मिके राज्ये सुभिक्षे निरुपद्रवे ।
कृत्वा तत्रैकं कुटीरं प्राचीरैः परिवेष्ठयेत् ॥ 5

In a good, devout kingdom where alms are easily available
and which is free from upheaval, build a hut and encircle
it with a wall.

वापीकूपतडागं च प्राचीरमध्यवर्ति च ।
नात्युच्चं नातिनिम्नं च कुटीरं कीटवर्जितम् ॥ 6

There should be a tank, a well, or a pond in the compound
and the hut should be neither too high nor too low and
free from insects.

सम्यग्गोमयलिप्तं च कुटीरं रन्ध्रवर्जितम् ।
एवं स्थाने हि गुप्ते च प्राणायामं समभ्यसेत् ॥ 7

The hut should be properly coated with cow dung and
free from holes. Only in a secluded place like that should
one practice pranayama.

हेमन्ते शिशिरे ग्रीष्मे वर्षायां च ऋतौ तथा ।
योगारम्भं न कुर्वीत कृते योगो हि रोगदः ॥ ८

Do not start a Yoga practice in winter, in the cool season, in summer, or during the rains. Started then, Yoga only brings illness.

वसन्ते शरदि प्रोक्तं योगारम्भं समाचरेत् ।
तदा योगो भवेत्सिद्धो रोगान्मुक्तो भवेद्ध्रुवम् ॥ ९

It is said that one should start to practice Yoga in spring or autumn. At those times Yoga is successful and one is sure to be freed from disease.

चैत्रादिफाल्गुनान्ते च माघादिफाल्गुनान्तिके ।
द्वौ द्वौ मासावृतुभागावनुभावश्चतुश्चतुः ॥ १०

There are two divisions of the seasons: into pairs of months, starting with Chaitra and ending in Phalguna, or into fours, according to when they are experienced, starting with Magha and ending in Phalguna.

वसन्तश्चैत्रवैशाखौ ज्येष्ठाषाढौ च ग्रीष्मकौ ।
वर्षा श्रावणभाद्राभ्यां शरदाश्विनकार्तिकौ ।
मार्गपौषौ च हेमन्तः शिशिरो माघफाल्गुनौ ॥ ११

Spring is Chaitra and Vaishakha, summer is Jyeshtha and Ashadha, the rains are Shravana and Bhadrapada, autumn

is Ashvina and Kartika, winter is Margashirsha and
Pausha, and the cool season is Magha and Phalguna.

अनुभावं प्रवक्ष्यामि ऋतूनां च यथोदितम् ।
माघादिमाधवान्तेषु वसन्तानुभवं विदुः ॥ 12

I shall teach when the seasons are said to be experienced.
They say spring is experienced from Margashirsha
to Vaishakha.

चैत्रादि चाषाढान्तं च निदाघानुभवं विदुः ।
आषाढादि चाश्विनान्तं प्रावृषानुभवं विदुः ॥ 13

They say that summer is experienced from Chaitra to
Ashadha, and the rains from Ashadha to Ashvina.

भाद्रादि मार्गशीर्षान्तं शरदोऽनुभवं विदुः ।
कार्तिकादिमाघमासान्तं हेमन्तानुभवं विदुः ।
मार्गादींश्चतुरो मासाञ्छिशिरानुभवं विदुः ॥ 14

They say that autumn is experienced from Bhadrapada to
Margashirsha, winter from Kartika to Magha, and the cool
season in the four months starting with Margashirsha.

वसन्ते वापि शरदि योगारम्भं तु समाचरेत् ।
तदा योगो भवेत्सिद्धो विनायासेन कथ्यते ॥ 15

Should the yogi start his Yoga practice in spring or autumn, then it is said that the Yoga will easily be successful.

मिताहारं विना यस्तु योगारम्भं तु कारयेत् ।
नानारोगो भवेत्तस्य किंचिद्योगो न सिध्यति ॥ 16

Should the yogi undertake the practice of Yoga without having a measured diet, he will get several diseases and his Yoga will in no way be successful.

शाल्यन्नं यवपिष्टं वा तथा गोधूमपिष्टकम् ।
मुद्नं माषचणकादि शुभ्रं च तुषवर्जितम् ॥ 17
पटोलं सुरणं मानं कक्कोलं च शुकाशकम् ।
द्राढिकां कर्कटीं रम्भां डुम्बरीं कण्टकण्टकम् ॥ 18
आमरम्भां बालरम्भां रम्भादण्डं च मूलकम् ।
वार्ताकिं मूलकमृद्धिं योगी भक्षणमाचरेत् ॥ 19

The yogi should eat rice, barley meal, wheat flour, and beans such as mung, urad, and chickpeas, all clean and without husks; parvar, yam, sago, kakkola berry, Indian trumpet, dradhika, long melon, plantain, dumbari, small eggplant, raw plantain, young plantain, plantain stalk and root, large eggplant, radish, and riddhi.

बालशाकं कालशाकं तथा पटोलपत्रकम् ।
पञ्चशाकं प्रशंसीयाद्वास्तुकं हिलमोचिकां ॥ 20

He should value the five leafy greens: amaranth leaf, holy basil, parvar leaf, lamb's quarters, and brahmi.

शुद्धं सुमधुरं स्निग्धमुदरार्धविवर्जितम् ।
भुज्यते सुरसंप्रीत्या मिताहारमिमं विदुः ॥ 21

A measured diet is said to consist of food that is pure, sweet, rich, leaves half the stomach empty, and is eaten with love for the gods.

अन्नेन पूरयेदर्धं तोयेन तु तृतीयकम् ।
उदरस्य तुरीयांशं संरक्षेद्वायुचारणे ॥ 22

One should fill half the stomach with food, a quarter with water, and leave the fourth quarter for the movement of air.

कट्वम्लं लवणं तिक्तं भृष्टं च दधि तक्रकम् ।
शाकोत्कटं तथा मद्यं तालं च पनसं तथा ॥ 23
कुलत्थं मसुरं पाण्डुं कूष्माण्डं शाकदण्डकम् ।
तुम्बीकोलकपित्थं च कण्टबिल्वं पलाशकम् ॥ 24
कदम्बं जम्बीरं बिम्बं लकुचं लशुनं विषम् ।
कामरङ्गं पियालं च हिङ्गुशाल्मलिकेमुकम् ॥ 25
योगारम्भे वर्जयेच्च पथिस्त्रीवह्निसेवनम् ॥ 26

Food that is pungent, sour, salty, bitter, or parched; curd, buttermilk, an excess of leafy greens, alcohol, palm nut, jackfruit, horse gram, masur and white beans, white pumpkin, the stalks of leafy greens, bottle gourd, jujube, elephant apple, thorny bel, dhak, kadamba, lemon, bimba, breadfruit, garlic, lotus stalk, wild turmeric, chironji, asafetida, the fruit of the silk-cotton tree, and taro root: these should be avoided by the yogi at the beginning of his Yoga practice, together with traveling, the company of women, and the use of fire.

नवनीतं घृतं क्षीरं शर्कराद्यैक्षवं गुडम् ।
पक्वरम्भां नारिकेलं दाडिम्बमशिवासवम् ।
द्राक्षां तु लवलीं धात्रीं रसमम्लविवर्जितम् ॥ 27
एलाजातिलवङ्गं च पौरुषं जम्बुजाम्बलम् ।
हरीतकीं च खर्जूरं योगी भक्षणमाचरेत् ॥ 28

Fresh butter, ghee, milk, sugar, sugarcane, jaggery, and so forth; ripe plantain, coconut, pomegranate, anise cordial, grapes, country gooseberry, amla fruit, juice that is not sour, cardamom, nutmeg, clove, paurusha, rose apple, haritaki, dates: the yogi should eat these.

लघुपाकं प्रियं स्निग्धं तथा धातुप्रपोषणम् ।
मनोभिलषितं योग्यं योगी भोजनमाचरेत् ॥ 29

The yogi should eat food which is easily digested, agreeable, and rich, which nourishes the body's constituents, which he wants to eat, and which is suitable.

कठिनं दुरितं पूतिमुष्णं पर्युषितं तथा ।
अतिशीतं चाति चोष्णं भक्ष्यं योगी विवर्जयेत् ॥ 30

The yogi should avoid food that is tough, off, putrid, sharp, stale, too cold, or too hot.

प्रातःस्नानोपवासादिकायक्लेशविधिं तथा ।
एकाहारं निशाहारं यामान्ते च न कारयेत् ॥ 31

He should not practice observances that harm the body, such as bathing in the early morning and fasting, nor should he eat only once a day, nor eat at night, nor at the end of the night.

एवंविधिविधानेन प्राणायामं समाचरेत् ।
आरम्भे प्रथमे कुर्यात्क्षीराज्यं नित्यभोजनम् ।
मध्याह्ने चैव सायाह्ने भोजनद्वयमाचरेत् ॥ 32

Following these rules, the yogi should practice pranayama. At the very beginning he should consume milk and ghee every day and take meals twice a day, at noon and in the evening.

कुशासने मृगाजिने व्याघ्राजिने च कम्बले ।
स्थूलासने समासीनः प्राङ्मुखो वाप्युदङ्मुखः ।
नाडीशुद्धिं समासाद्य प्राणायामं समभ्यसेत् ॥ 33

Sitting on a thick seat made of either kusha grass, an antelope skin, a tiger skin, or a blanket, he should cleanse his nadis and then practice pranayama."

नाडीशुद्धिं कथं कुर्यान्नाडीशुद्धिस्तु कीदृशी ।
तत्सर्वं श्रोतुमिच्छामि तद्वदस्व दयानिधे ॥ 34

Chanda the Skullbearer said, "I want to hear all about how one might cleanse the nadis and what their purification is like. So tell me, O treasury of compassion."

मलाकुलासु नाडीषु मारुतो नैव गच्छति ।
प्राणायामः कथं सिध्येत्तत्त्वज्ञानं कथं भवेत् ।
तस्मान्नाडीशुद्धिमादौ प्राणायामं ततोऽभ्यसेत् ॥ 35

Gheranda replied, "The wind cannot flow through nadis clogged with dirt. How could pranayama succeed? How could knowledge of Reality arise? Therefore the yogi should first purify the nadis and then practice pranayama.

नाडीशुद्धिर्द्विधा प्रोक्ता समनुर्निर्मनुस्तथा ।
बीजेन समनुं कुर्यान्निर्मनुं धौतिकर्मणा ॥ 36

The purification of the nadis is said to be of two kinds: Samanu and Nirmanu. The yogi should do Samanu by means of a seed mantra and Nirmanu by means of the dhauti cleansing practices.

धौतिकर्म पुरा प्रोक्तं षड्कर्मसाधने यथा ।
शृणुष्व समनुं चण्ड नाडीशुद्धिर्यथा भवेत् ॥ 37

The dhauti cleansing practices have already been taught in the section on how to master the six cleansing techniques, so, Chanda, hear about Samanu, by which the nadis can be purified.

उपविश्यासने योगी पद्मासनं समाचरेत् ।
गुर्वादिन्यासनं कृत्वा यथैव गुरुभाषितम् ।
नाडीशुद्धिं प्रकुर्वीत प्राणायामविशुद्धये ॥ 38

The yogi should sit on his seat and assume Padmasana. After ritually installing his guru and so forth in his body as taught by his guru, he should purify his nadis so that he might be completely pure for pranayama.

वायुबीजं ततो ध्यात्वा धूम्रवर्णं सतेजसम् ।
चन्द्रेण पूरयेद्वायुं बीजषोडशकैः सुधीः ॥ 39

The wise yogi should meditate upon the seed mantra of the wind as smoke colored and shiny, then inhale air through the lunar channel, repeating the seed mantra sixteen times.[1]

चतुःषष्ट्या मात्रया च कुम्भकेनैव धारयेत् ।
द्वात्रिंशन्मात्रया वायुं सूर्यनाड्या च रेचयेत् ॥ 40

Using kumbhaka, he should hold the air for sixty-four repetitions and exhale it through the solar channel for thirty-two repetitions.

---

[1]The seed mantra of the wind is said to be *ya* in verse 3.62. The lunar channel (Ida) starts at the left nostril, the solar channel (Pingala) at the right.

उत्थाप्याग्निं नाभिमूलाद्ध्यायेत्तेजोऽवनीयुतम् ।
वह्निबीजषोडशेन सूर्यनाड्या च पूरयेत् ॥ 41

Having raised fire from the base of the navel, he should
meditate on it as being joined with earth. He should
inhale through the solar channel for sixteen repetitions of
the seed mantra of fire.

चतुःषष्ट्या मात्रया च कुम्भकेनैव धारयेत् ।
द्वात्रिंशन्मात्रया वायुं शशिनाड्या च रेचयेत् ॥ 42

Using kumbhaka, he should hold the air for sixty-four
repetitions and exhale it through the lunar channel for
thirty-two repetitions.

नासाग्रे शशधृग्बिम्बं ध्यात्वा ज्योत्स्नासमन्वितम् ।
ठंबीजषोडशेनैव इडया पूरयेन्मरुत् ॥ 43

Meditating on the shining orb of the moon at the tip of
the nose, he should inhale through Ida for sixteen repetitions of the seed mantra *tham*.

चतुःषष्ट्या मात्रया च वंबीजेनैव धारयेत् ।
अमृतप्लावितं ध्यात्वा नाडीधौतिं विभावयेत्
द्वात्रिंशेन लकारेण दृढं भाव्यं विरेचयेत् ॥ 44

He should hold his breath for sixty-four repetitions of the
seed mantra *vam*. Meditating on himself as being flooded
with the nectar of immortality, he should imagine his

nadis being bathed. Keeping his visualization steady, he should exhale for thirty-two repetitions of *la*.

एवंविधां नाडीशुद्धिं कृत्वा नाडीं विशोधयेत् ।
दृढो भूत्वासनं कृत्वा प्राणायामं समाचरेत् ॥ 45

He should purify his nadis by means of this nadi purification technique. Fixing himself firmly in an asana, he should then perform pranayama.

सहितः सूर्यभेदश्च उज्जायी शीतली तथा ।
भस्त्रिका भ्रामरी मूर्च्छा केवली चाष्ट कुम्भकाः ॥ 46

Sahita, Suryabheda, Ujjayi, Shitali, Bhastrika, Bhramari, Murccha, and Kevali are the eight kumbhakas.

सहितो द्विविधः प्रोक्तः सगर्भश्च निगर्भकः ।
सगर्भो बीजमुच्चार्य निगर्भो बीजवर्जितः ॥ 47

Sahita is said to be of two kinds: seeded and unseeded. When it is seeded, the seed mantra is repeated; when it is unseeded, it is without a seed mantra.

प्राणायामं सगर्भं च प्रथमं कथयामि ते ।
सुखासने चोपविश्य प्राङ्मुखो वाप्युदङ्मुखः ।
रजोगुणं विधिं ध्यायेद्रक्तवर्णमवर्णकम् ॥ 48

I shall teach you the seeded pranayama first. Sitting in a comfortable asana and facing east or north, the yogi should meditate on Brahma the Creator as having the quality rajas, the color red, and the letter *a*.

इडया पूरयेद्वायुं मात्रया षोडशैः सुधीः ।
पूरकान्ते कुम्भकाद्ये कर्तव्यस्तूड्डीयानकः ॥ 49

The wise yogi should inhale through Ida for sixteen repetitions. Uddiyana is to be performed at the end of the inhalation and the start of kumbhaka.

सत्त्वमयं हरिं ध्यात्वा उकारं कृष्णवर्णकम् ।
चतुःषष्ट्या च मात्रया कुम्भकेनैव धारयेत् ॥ 50

He should meditate on Vishnu as having the quality sattva, the letter *u*, and the color black, and hold his breath by means of kumbhaka for sixty-four repetitions.

तमोमयं शिवं ध्यात्वा मकारं शुक्रवर्णकम् ।
द्वात्रिंशन्मात्रया चैव रेचयेद्रविणा पुनः ॥ 51

He should meditate on Shiva as having the quality tamas, the letter *ma*, and the color white, and then exhale through the solar channel for thirty-two repetitions.[2]

---

[2]When combined, the letters associated with the three deities make *om*.

पुनः पिङ्गलयापूर्य कुम्भकेनैव धारयेत् ।
इडया रेचयेत्पश्चात्तद्वीजेन क्रमेण तु ॥ 52

After then inhaling through Pingala, he should hold
his breath by means of kumbhaka before proceeding to
exhale through Ida with the seed mantra.

अनुलोमविलोमेन वारं वारं च साधयेत् ।
पूरकान्ते कुम्भकान्तं धृतनासापुटद्वयम् ।
कनिष्ठानामिकाङ्गुष्ठैस्तर्जनीमध्यमे विना ॥ 53

Changing from side to side, he should practice over and
over again. From the end of the inhalation to the end
of kumbhaka, both nostrils should be held by the little
finger, the ring finger, and the thumb, without the index
and middle fingers.

प्राणायामो निगर्भस्तु विना बीजेन जायते ।
वामजानूपरिन्यस्तं वामपाणितलं भ्रमेत् ।
एकादिशतपर्यन्तं पूरकुम्भकरेचनम् ॥ 54

The seedless pranayama takes place without a seed
mantra. The yogi should place the palm of his left hand
above his left knee and move it around in a circle. Inhalation, kumbhaka, and exhalation start at the first rotation
and finish with the hundredth.

उत्तमा विंशतिर्मात्रा मध्यमा षोडशी स्मृता ।

अधमा द्वादशी मात्रा प्राणायामास्त्रिधा स्मृताः ॥ 55

Three types of pranayama are taught: the highest has an inhalation of twenty units, in the middle pranayama it lasts sixteen units, and in the lowest, twelve.

अधमाज्जायते घर्मो मेरुकम्पश्च मध्यमात् ।
उत्तमाच भूमित्यागस्त्रिविधं सिद्धिलक्षणम् ॥ 56

The signs of success are threefold: in the lowest, heat is produced; in the middle, the spine shakes; and in the highest, the yogi leaves the ground.

प्राणायामात्खेचरत्वं प्राणायामादुजां हतिः ।
प्राणायामाच्छक्तिबोधः प्राणायामान्मनोन्मनी ।
आनन्दो जायते चित्ते प्राणायामी सुखी भवेत् ॥ 57

Through pranayama, the yogi gets the ability to move through space; through pranayama, diseases are destroyed; through pranayama, Shakti is awakened; through pranayama, manonmani arises. Bliss arises in the mind and the practitioner of pranayama becomes happy.

कथितं सहितं कुम्भं सूर्यभेदनकं शृणु ।
पूरयेत्सूर्यनाड्या च यथाशक्ति बहिर्मरुत् ॥ 58

Sahitakumbhaka has been taught. Now hear about Suryabheda. Inhale through the solar channel as much external air as possible.

धारयेद्दृढयत्नेन कुम्भकेन जलन्धरैः ।
यावत्स्वेदं नखकेशाभ्यां तावत्कुर्वन्तु कुम्भकम् ॥ 59

Using kumbhaka and Jalandhara, make great efforts to hold the breath. Yogis should do kumbhaka until there is sweat in their nails and hair.

प्राणोऽपानः समानश्चोदानव्यानौ तथैव च ।
सर्वे ते सूर्यसंभिन्ना नाभिमूलात्समुद्धरेत् ॥ 60

Prana, apana, samana, udana, and vyana: they are all connected to the sun. Raise them from the navel.[3]

इडया रेचयेत्पश्चाद्धैर्येणाखण्डवेगतः ।
पुनः सूर्येण चाकृष्य कुम्भयित्वा यथाविधि ॥ 61

Then exhale through Ida, steadily and without interrupting the flow. Next inhale through the solar channel and hold the breath with kumbhaka as prescribed.

रेचयित्वा साधयेत्तु क्रमेण च पुनः पुनः ।
कुम्भकः सूर्यभेदस्तु जरामृत्युविनाशकः ॥ 62

After exhaling, practice in sequence over and over again. The Suryabheda kumbhaka destroys decrepitude and death.

---

[3]These are the five vital airs that animate the body. According to Gorakhnath in the *Goraksha Samhita*, verses 34–35, prana inhabits the region of the heart, apana that of the anus, samana the navel, udana the throat, and vyana pervades the whole body.

बोधयेत्कुण्डलीं शक्तिं देहाग्निं च विवर्धयेत् ।
इति ते कथितं चण्ड सूर्यभेदनमुत्तमम् ॥ 63

It awakens Kundalini Shakti and increases the bodily
fire. You have thus been taught the lofty Suryabheda,
O Chanda.

नासाभ्यां वायुमाकृष्य मुखमध्ये च धारयेत् ।
हृत्तलाभ्यां समाकृष्य वायुं वक्त्रे च धारयेत् ॥ 64

Draw in air through both nostrils and hold it in the
mouth. After drawing it through the chest and throat,
hold it in the mouth again.

मुखं प्रक्षाल्य संवन्द्य कुर्याज्जालन्धरं ततः ।
आशक्ति कुम्भकं कृत्वा धारयेदविरोधतः ॥ 65

After rinsing the air around the mouth, bow the head,
perform Jalandhara, and hold the breath for as long
as is comfortable.

उज्ज्ञायीकुम्भकं कृत्वा सर्वकार्याणि साधयेत् ।
न भवेत्कफरोगश्च क्रूरवायुरजीर्णकम् ॥ 66

After performing the Ujjayi kumbhaka, the yogi can
succeed in everything he does. Diseases of kapha do not
arise, nor problems with wind, nor indigestion.

आमवातः क्षयः कासो ज्वरः प्लीहा न जायते ।
जरामृत्युविनाशाय चोज्ज्ञायीं साधयेन्नरः ॥ 67

Constipation, consumption, cough, fever, and disorders of
the spleen do not arise. To destroy decrepitude and death
a man should master Ujjayi.

जिह्वया वायुमाकृष्य उदरे पूरयेच्छनैः ।
क्षणं च कुम्भकं कृत्वा नासाभ्यां रेचयेत्पुनः ॥ 68

Inhale slowly, drawing air through the tongue into the
stomach. After briefly performing kumbhaka, exhale
through the nostrils.

सर्वदा साधयेद्योगी शीतलीकुम्भकं शुभम् ।
अजीर्णं कफपित्तं च नैव तस्य प्रजायते ॥ 69

Regularly practice Shitalikumbhaka; it is beneficial. One
gets neither indigestion nor disorders of kapha and pitta.

भस्त्रिका लोहकाराणां यथा क्रमेण संभ्रमेत् ।
तथा वायुं च नासाभ्यामुभाभ्यां चालयेच्छनैः ॥ 70

Slowly move air through the nostrils in the same way that
a blacksmith's bellows successively opens and closes.

एवं विंशतिवारं च कृत्वा कुर्याच्च कुम्भकम् ।
तदन्ते चालयेद्वायुं पूर्वोक्तं च यथाविधि ॥ 71

After doing this twenty times, perform kumbhaka. At its end, exhale in the manner described earlier.

त्रिवारं साधयेदेनं भस्त्रिकाकुम्भकं सुधीः ।
न च रोगो न च क्लेश आरोग्यं च दिने दिने ॥ 72

The wise yogi should practice this Bhastrikakumbhaka three times. He will have neither illness nor distress and will become healthier every day.

अर्धरात्रे गते योगी जन्तुशब्दविवर्जिते ।
कर्णौ पिधाय हस्ताभ्यां कुर्यात्पूरककुम्भकम् ॥ 73

At midnight in a place free from animals and noise, block the ears with the hands, inhale, and perform kumbhaka.

श‍ृणुयाद्दक्षिणे कर्णे नादमन्तर्गतं सुधीः ।
प्रथमं झिल्लिकानादं वंशीनादं ततः परम् ॥ 74

The wise yogi should hear the internal sound in his right ear. At first it is the sound of a cricket, then that of a bamboo flute.

मेघझर्झरभ्रमरी घण्टा कांस्यं ततः परम् ।
तुरीभेरीमृदङ्गादिनिनादानेकदुन्दुभिः ॥ 75

Then it is thunder, a jharjhara drum, a bee, a bell, and a gong, followed by the sounds of a trumpet, a kettledrum, a tabor, and so forth, and several dundubhi drums.

एवं नानाविधो नादो जायते नित्यमभ्यसात् ।
अनाहतस्य शब्दस्य तस्य शब्दस्य यो ध्वनिः ॥ 76

Various sounds like these arise through regular practice of
the unstruck sound. That sound has a resonance.

ध्वनेरन्तर्गतं ज्योतिर्ज्योतिरन्तर्गतं मनः ।
तन्मनो विलयं याति तद्विष्णोः परमं पदम् ।
एवं भ्रामरीसंसिद्धिः समाधिसिद्धिमाप्नुयात् ॥ 77

In the resonance is a light and in the light is the mind. In
it the mind attains absorption. That is the ultimate seat
of Vishnu. Thus there is success in Bhramari and the yogi
may achieve success in samadhi.

सुखेन कुम्भकं कृत्वा मनश्च भ्रुवोरन्तरम् ।
संत्यज्य विषयान्सर्वान्मनोमूर्च्छा सुखप्रदा ।
आत्मनि मनसो योगादानन्दं जायते ध्रुवम् ॥ 78

By performing kumbhaka without straining, placing the
mind between the eyebrows, and abandoning all objects,
the mind enters an agreeable trance. By joining the mind
to the self, bliss is sure to arise.

हंकारेण बहिर्याति सःकारेण विशेत्पुनः ।
षट्शतानि दिवारात्रौ सहस्राण्येकविंशतिः ।
अजपां नाम गायत्रीं जीवो जपति सर्वदा ॥ 79

In a day and a night the breath goes out with the sound *ham* and comes back in with the sound *sa* 21,600 times. The jiva constantly repeats this Gayatri called Ajapa.[4]

मूलाधारे यथा हंसस्तथा हि हृदि पङ्कजे ।
तथा नासापुटद्वन्द्वे त्रिभिर्हंससमागमः ॥ 80

Just as the hamsa is in the Muladhara, so is it in the lotus in the heart and the two nostrils. Hamsa comes together by way of these three places.[5]

षण्णवत्यङ्गुलीमानं शरीरं कर्मरूपकम् ।
देहाद्बहिर्गतो वायुः स्वभावाद्द्वादशाङ्गुलिः ॥ 81

The body is formed by its actions and measures ninety-six fingerwidths. In the natural state, when air goes out of the body it travels twelve fingers.

गायने षोडशाङ्गुल्यो भोजने विंशतिस्तथा ।
चतुर्विंशाङ्गुलिः पन्थे निद्रायां त्रिंशदङ्गुलिः ।
मैथुने षट्त्रिंशदुक्तं व्यायामे च ततोऽधिकम् ॥ 82

When one sings, it travels sixteen fingers and when one eats, twenty. When one walks, it travels twenty-four

---

[4]The Gayatri is a twenty-four-syllable Vedic hymn that every Brahmin should recite daily. Here Gheranda is teaching the yogic alternative. Ajapa literally means "unpronounced."

[5]Hamsa (literally "swan") is the union of the out- and inbreaths.

fingers; in sleep, thirty fingers. During sex it is said
to travel thirty-six fingers and during exercise it goes
further still.

स्वभावेऽस्य गतेर्न्यूने परमायुः प्रवर्धति ।
आयुःक्षयोऽधिके प्रोक्तो मारुते चान्तराग्नते ॥ 83

When its natural range decreases, then life is lengthened.
Life is said to shorten when the air coming from within
travels further.

तस्मात्प्राणे स्थिते देहे मरणं नैव जायते ।
वायुना घटसंबन्धे भवेत्केवलकुम्भकः ॥ 84

Thus when the breath is in the body death cannot occur.
When air is confined in the body there is Kevalakumbhaka.

यावज्जीवं जपेन्मन्त्रमजपासंख्यकेवलम् ।
अद्यावधि धृतं संख्याविभ्रमं केवलीकृते ॥ 85

While he is alive the yogi should recite the mantra.
Kevala has the frequency of Ajapa. When Kevala is
performed, if it is held for too long the rate is disrupted.

अत एव हि कर्तव्यः केवलीकुम्भको नरैः ।
केवली चाजपासंख्या द्विगुणा च मनोन्मनी ॥ 86

For this reason alone men should perform Kevalakumbhaka. Kevala is at the Ajapa frequency; manonmani
is twice that.

नासाभ्यां वायुमाकृष्य केवलं कुम्भकं चरेत् ।
एकादिकचतुःषष्टिं धारयेत्प्रथमे दिने ॥ 87

Draw in air through the nostrils and perform Kevalakumbhaka. On the first day hold it from one to sixty-four times.

केवलीमष्टधा कुर्याद्यामे यामे दिने दिने ।
अथवा पञ्चधा कुर्याद्यथा तत्कथयामि ते ॥ 88

Do it eight times a day, every three hours, or do it five
times a day in the manner that I shall tell you.

प्रातर्मध्याह्नसायाह्ने मध्यरात्रे चतुर्थके ।
त्रिसंध्यमथ वा कुर्यात्सममाने दिने दिने ॥ 89

Do it in the morning, at noon, in the evening, at
midnight, and in the fourth watch of the night.
Otherwise do it at the three junctures in equal intervals
every day.[6]

पञ्चवारं दिने वृद्धिवरिकं च दिने तथा ।

---

[6]That is, at four o'clock in the morning, at noon, and at eight o'clock in
the evening.

अजपापरिमाणं च यावत्सिद्धिः प्रजायते ॥ 90

The length of Ajapa should be increased every day from one to five times until success arises.

प्राणायामं केवलीं च तदा वदति योगवित् ।
केवलीकुम्भके सिद्धे किं न सिध्यति भूतले ॥ 91

The knower of Yoga then calls pranayama Kevala. When Kevalakumbhaka is perfected there is nothing on earth that cannot be accomplished.

इति श्रीघेरण्डसंहितायां घेरण्डचण्डसंवादे
घटस्थयोगप्रकरणे प्राणायामप्रयोगो नाम पञ्चमोपदेशः ॥

Thus ends the fifth chapter, called the practice of pranayama, in the glorious Gheranda Samhita, a dialogue between Gheranda and Chanda and a treatise on bodily Yoga.

Chapter Six

Dhyana

स्थूलं ज्योतिस्तथा सूक्ष्मं ध्यानस्य त्रिविधं विदुः ।
स्थूलं मूर्तिमयं प्रोक्तं ज्योतिस्तेजोमयं तथा ।
सूक्ष्मं बिन्दुमयं ब्रह्म कुण्डली परदेवता ॥ १

There are said to be three types of dhyana: gross, luminous, and subtle. Gross is of an image and luminous is of light. Subtle dhyana is of bindu. It is Brahman, and Kundalini is the ultimate deity.

स्वकीयहृदये ध्यायेत्सुधासागरमुत्तमम् ।
तन्मध्ये रत्नद्वीपं तु सुरत्नवालुकामयम् ॥ २

The yogi should visualize a sublime ocean of nectar in his heart, with an island of jewels in its middle whose sand is made of gemstones.

चतुर्दिक्षु नीपतरुं बहुपुष्पसमन्वितम् ।
नीपोपवनसंकुलैर्वेष्टितं परिखा इव ॥ ३
मालतीमल्लिकाजातीकेसरैश्चम्पकैस्तथा ।

पारिजातैः स्थलपद्मैर्गन्धामोदितदिङ्मुखैः ॥ ४

In every direction there are kadamba trees with abundant flowers and it is ringed with a thick kadamba forest like a stockade, where the scents of malati, mallika, jati, kaisara, champa, parijata, and sthalapadma flowers perfume every quarter.

तन्मध्ये संस्मरेद्योगी कल्पीवृक्षं मनोहरम् ।
चतुःशाखाचतुर्वेदं नित्यपुष्पफलान्वितम् ॥ ५

In its middle the yogi should imagine an enchanting, wish-fulfilling tree whose four branches are the four Vedas and which permanently bears flowers and fruit.

भ्रमराः कोकिलास्तत्र गुञ्जन्ति निगदन्ति च ।
ध्यायेत्तत्र स्थिरो भूत्वा महामाणिक्यमण्डपम् ॥ ६

Bees and cuckoos buzz and call there. He should steady himself and visualize a great jeweled pavilion there.

तन्मध्ये तु स्मरेद्योगी पर्यङ्कं सुमनोहरम् ।
तत्रेष्टदेवतां ध्यायेद्यद्ध्यानं गुरुभाषितम् ॥ ७

In its middle he should imagine a delightful throne on which he should visualize his tutelary deity according to the dhyana taught by his guru.

यस्य देवस्य यद्रूपं यथा भूषणवाहनम् ।
तद्रूपं ध्यायते नित्यं स्थूलध्यानमिदं विदुः ॥ 8

That deity should regularly be meditated upon with its associated form, ornaments, and vehicle. This is called gross dhyana.

सहस्रारे महापद्मे कर्णिकायां विचिन्तयेत् ।
विलग्नसहितं पद्मं दलैर्द्वादशभिर्युतम् ॥ 9

The yogi should visualize a lotus attached to the pericarp of the great thousand-petaled lotus.

शुक्लवर्णं महातेजो द्वादशैर्बीजभाषितम् ।
हसक्षमलवरयुंहसखफ्रें यथाक्रमम् ॥ 10

It is white, luminous, and has twelve seed syllables: *ha, sa, ksha, ma, la, va, ra, yum, ha, sa, kha,* and *phrem,* in that order.

तन्मध्ये कर्णिकायां तु अकथादिरेखात्रयम् ।
हलक्षकोणसंयुक्तं प्रणवं तत्र वर्तते ॥ 11

In the middle of its pericarp is a triangle made of the syllables *a, ka, tha,* and so forth, at whose corners are *ha, la,* and *ksha.* Inside it is *om.*

नादबिन्दुमयं पीठं ध्यायेत्तत्र मनोहरम् ।

तत्रोपरि हंसयुग्मं पादुका तत्र वर्तते ॥ 12

The yogi should imagine a beautiful seat there consisting
of nada and bindu. On it are a pair of swans and a pair
of wooden sandals.

ध्यायेत्तत्र गुरुं देवं द्विभुजं च त्रिलोचनम् ।
श्वेताम्बरधरं देवं शुक्रगन्धानुलेपनम् ॥ 13
शुक्रपुष्पमयं माल्यं रक्तशक्तिसमन्वितम् ।
एवंविधगुरुध्यानात्स्थूलध्यानं प्रसिध्यति ॥ 14

He should visualize his guru there as a god with two
arms and three eyes, dressed in white, bedaubed with
white-scented paste, wearing a garland of white flowers,
and in the company of his crimson Shakti. By dhyana of
the guru like this, the gross dhyana is perfected.

स्थूलध्यानं तु कथितं तेजोध्यानं शृणुष्व मे ।
यद्ध्यानेन योगसिद्धिरात्मप्रत्यक्षमेव च ॥ 15

I have described the gross dhyana. Hear from me the
luminous dhyana, by which Yoga is perfected and the soul
is directly perceived.

मूलाधारे कुण्डलिनी भुजगाकाररूपिणी ।
तत्र तिष्ठति जीवात्मा प्रदीपकलिकाकृतिः ।
ध्यायेत्तेजोमयं ब्रह्म तेजोध्यानं परात्परम् ॥ 16

Kundalini is in the Muladhara in the form of a snake. The jivatman dwells there in the form of the flame of a lamp. Meditate on Brahman as made of light. This is the supreme, luminous dhyana.

भ्रुवोर्मध्ये मनऊर्ध्वे यत्तेजः प्रणवात्मकम् ।
ध्यायेज्ज्वालावलीयुक्तं तेजोध्यानं तदेव हि ॥ 17

Between the eyebrows and above the mind is a light consisting of *om*. Meditate on it as joined with a ring of fire. That is the luminous dhyana.

तेजोध्यानं श्रुतं चण्ड सूक्ष्मध्यानं वदाम्यहम् ।
बहुभाग्यवशाद्यस्य कुण्डली जाग्रती भवेत् ॥ 18
आत्मना सह योगेन नेत्ररन्ध्रादिनिर्गता ।
विहरेद्राजमार्गे च चञ्चलत्वान्न दृश्यते ॥ 19

You have heard the luminous dhyana, Chanda; I shall describe the subtle dhyana. When through abundant good fortune the yogi's Kundalini awakens, she joins with the self, exits through the sockets of the eyes, and roams about the royal road. Because she flits about, she cannot be seen.

शाम्भवीमुद्रया योगी ध्यानयोगेन सिध्यति ।
सूक्ष्मध्यानमिदं गोप्यं देवानामपि दुर्लभम् ॥ 20

The yogi attains success through Shambhavimudra and dhyana Yoga. This subtle dhyana is to be kept secret. It is hard for even the gods to attain.

स्थूलध्यानाच्छतगुणं तेजोध्यानं प्रचक्षते ।
तेजोध्यानाल्लक्षगुणं सूक्ष्मध्यानं परात्परम् ॥ 21

The luminous dhyana is considered to be a hundred times better than the gross dhyana, and the supreme, subtle dhyana is a hundred thousand times better than the luminous dhyana.

इति ते कथितं चण्ड ध्यानयोगं सुदुर्लभम् ।
आत्मा साक्षाद्भवेद्यस्मात्तस्माद्ध्यानं विशिष्यते ॥ 22

Thus have I taught you the very precious dhyana Yoga. By means of it, the soul becomes directly perceptible. That is why dhyana is special.

इति श्रीघेरण्डसंहितायां घेरण्डचण्डसंवादे
घटस्थयोगे सप्तसाधने ध्यानयोगो नाम षष्ठोपदेशः ॥

Thus ends the sixth chapter, called dhyana Yoga, in the glorious Gheranda Samhita, a dialogue between Gheranda and Chanda on the seven means of bodily Yoga.

Samadhi

समाधिश्च परो योगो बहुभाग्येन लभ्यते ।
गुरोः कृपाप्रसादेन प्राप्यते गुरुभक्तितः ॥ 1

Samadhi, the highest Yoga, is attained by the very
fortunate. It is received through the compassion and
grace of the guru and by devotion to him.

विद्याप्रतीतिः स्वगुरुप्रतीतिरात्मप्रतीतिर्मनसः प्रबोधः ।
दिने दिने यस्य भवेत्स योगी सुशोभनाभ्यासमुपैति सद्यः ॥ 2

That yogi quickly attains the most beautiful practice who
every day has conviction in his learning, conviction in his
guru, conviction in his self, and awakening of his mind.

घटाङ्गिन्नं मनः कृत्वा चैक्यं कुर्यात्परात्मनि ।
समाधिं तं विजानीयान्मुक्तसंङ्गो दशादिभिः ॥ 3

Separate the mind from the body and unite it with the
supreme soul. When your consciousness is free from its
different states, know that to be samadhi.

अहं ब्रह्म न चान्योऽस्मि ब्रह्मैवाहं न शोकभाक् ।
सच्चिदानन्दरूपोऽहं नित्यमुक्तः स्वभाववान् ॥ ४

I am Brahman and nothing else. I am Brahman alone and
do not suffer. My form is truth, consciousness, and bliss.
I am eternally free. I abide in my own nature.

शाम्भव्या चैव भ्रामर्या खेचर्या योनिमुद्रया ।
ध्यानं नादं रसानन्दं लयसिद्धिश्चतुर्विधा ॥ ५

By means of Shambhavi, Bhramari, Khechari, and
Yonimudra, four types of samadhi arise: dhyana, nada,
rasananda, and laya siddhi.[1]

पञ्चधा भक्तियोगेन मनोमूर्च्छा च षड्विधा ।
षड्विधोऽयं राजयोगः प्रत्येकमवधारयेत् ॥ ६

The fifth is by means of devotion and the sixth is trance.
This is the sixfold Raja Yoga. Understand each of them.

शाम्भवीं मुद्रिकां कृत्वा आत्मप्रत्यक्षमानयेत् ।
बिन्दु ब्रह्ममयं दृष्ट्वा मनस्तत्र नियोजयेत् ॥ ७

Using Shambhavimudra, bring about perception of the
self. On seeing the bindu that consists of Brahman, fix
your mind there.

---

[1]Nada is sound, rasananda means "bliss in taste," and laya siddhi means "success
in absorption."

खमध्ये कुरु चात्मानमात्ममध्ये च खं कुरु ।
आत्मानं खमयं दृष्ट्वा न किंचिदपि बुध्यते ।
सदानन्दमयो भूत्वा समाधिस्थो भवेन्नरः ॥ ८

Put the self in space and space in the self. When one sees
the self as made of space, nothing else is perceived. When
a man consists of truth and bliss, he is in samadhi.

अनिलं मन्दवेगेन भ्रामरीकुम्भकं चरेत् ।
मन्दं मन्दं रेचयेद्वायुं भृङ्गनादं ततो भवेत् ॥ ९

Slowly draw in air and perform Bhramarikumbhaka.
Exhale it very slowly and then the sound of a bee will arise.

अन्तःस्थं भ्रमरीनादं श्रुत्वा तत्र मनो नयेत् ।
समाधिर्जायते तत्र चानन्दः सोऽहमित्यतः ॥ १०

On hearing the sound of a bee from within, lead the
mind there. Samadhi will occur, together with the bliss
arising from the realization, 'I am that.'

खेचरीमुद्रासाधनादूसनोर्ध्वगता यदा ।
तदा समाधिसिद्धिः स्याद्धित्वा साधारणक्रियाम् ॥ ११

When the tongue goes upwards in the practice of
Khecharimudra then samadhi is perfected without performing any of the ordinary practices.

योनिमुद्रां समासाद्य स्वयं शक्तिमयो भवेत् ।
सुशृङ्गाररसेनैव विहरेत्परमात्मनि ॥ 12

By performing Yonimudra, the yogi can himself become
one with Shakti. In the bliss of sexual love, he can sport
in the supreme self.

आनन्दमयः संभूत्वा ऐक्यं ब्रह्मणि संभवेत् ।
अहं ब्रह्मेति चाद्वैतसमाधिस्तेन जायते ॥ 13

Becoming one with bliss, he attains unity with Brahman.
By the realization that he is Brahman, nondual samadhi
arises.

स्वकीयहृदये ध्यायेदिष्टदेवस्वरूपकम् ।
चिन्तयेद्भक्तियोगेन परमाह्लादपूर्वकम् ॥ 14

In your heart visualize your tutelary deity. Contemplate it
with devotion and supreme joy.

आनन्दाश्रुपुलकेन दशाभावः प्रजायते ।
समाधिः संभवेत्तेन संभवेच्च मनोन्मनी ॥ 15

A condition arises that is accompanied by bliss, tears, and
goose bumps. Samadhi arises and manonmani follows
on from it.

मनोमूर्च्छां समासाद्य मन आत्मनि योजयेत् ।

परात्मनः समायोगात्समाधिं समवाप्नुयात् ॥ 16

Entrance your mind and insert it into the self. Through union with the highest self one can attain samadhi.

इति ते कथितं चण्ड समाधिर्मुक्तिलक्षणम् ।
राजयोगः समाधिः स्यादेकात्मन्येव साधनम् ।
उन्मनी सहजावस्था सर्वे चैकात्मवाचकाः ॥ 17

Chanda, I have thus taught you samadhi, which is characterized by liberation. Raja Yoga, or samadhi, is the means to union with the self. Together with unmani and sahajavastha, they are synonyms of union with the self.

जले विष्णुः स्थले विष्णुर्विष्णुः पर्वतमस्तके ।
ज्वालामालाकुले विष्णुः सर्वं विष्णुमयं जगत् ॥ 18

Vishnu is in the water, Vishnu is on the land, Vishnu is on the mountaintop, Vishnu is in the thick of the garland of flames. The entire universe consists of Vishnu.

भूचराः खेचराश्चामी यावन्तो जीवजन्तवः ।
वृक्षगुल्मलतावल्लीतृणाद्या वारि पर्वताः ।
सर्वं ब्रह्म विजानीयात्सर्वं पश्यति चात्मनि ॥ 19

All the creatures of the earth, all the creatures of the air, plants such as trees, shrubs, creepers, vines, grasses, water, and mountains: know all these to be Brahman and see them all in the self.

आत्मा घटस्थचैतन्यमद्वैतं शाश्वतं परम् ।
घटादिभिन्नतो ज्ञात्वा वीतरागं विवासनम् ॥ 20

In the body the self is consciousness. It is without a second, eternal and supreme. Because it is separate from the body, realize that you are free from passion and vices.

एवं मिथः समाधिः स्यात्सर्वसंकल्पवर्जितः ।
स्वदेहे पुत्रदारादिबान्धवेषु धनादिषु ।
सर्वेषु निर्ममो भूत्वा समाधिं समवाप्नुयात् ॥ 21

Thus samadhi is also free from all ideation. After becoming disinterested in one's body, one's children, one's wife, one's relatives, one's friends, riches, and everything else, one can attain samadhi.

तत्त्वं लयामृतं गोप्यं शिवोक्तं विविधानि च ।
तेषां संक्षेपमादाय कथितं मुक्तिलक्षणम् ॥ 22

The truth, the secret nectar of absorption, has been taught by Shiva along with various other subjects. I have taught you an abridgement of them, the aim of which is liberation.

इति ते कथितः चण्ड समाधिर्दुर्लभः परः ।
यं ज्ञात्वा न पुनर्जन्म जायते भूमिमण्डले ॥ 23

Chanda, I have thus taught you the precious, supreme
samadhi, by knowledge of which, rebirth on the earth
does not occur."

इति श्रीघेरण्डसंहितायां घेरण्डचण्डसंवादे घटस्थयोगसाधने
योगस्य सप्तसारे समाधियोगो नाम सप्तमोपदेशः समाप्तः ॥

Thus ends the seventh chapter, called samadhi Yoga, in
the glorious Gheranda Samhita, a dialogue between
Gheranda and Chanda on the yogic technique of bodily
Yoga which has seven essential parts.

Contributors

JAMES MALLINSON is a graduate of Eton and Oxford, holds a master's from the School of Oriental and African Studies, University of London, and returned to Oxford University for his doctorate. He has also spent years in India, living amongst the yogis.

SANTOSHA VANESSA BOUCHARD, the woman in the photographs, is a lifelong practitioner of Yoga.
She inspires her students through her love of Yoga.
Michael L. Rixson has been a professional photographer since 1983 and a practitioner of Yoga since 1997.

YOGAVIDYA.COM is dedicated to publishing excellent and affordable books about Yoga. It is completely independent of any commercial, governmental, educational, or religious institutions.

CPSIA information can be obtained
at www.ICGtesting.com
Printed in the USA
BVHW07s1211200518
516784BV00001B/80/P